KU-497-940

A NURSE'S SURVIVAL GUIDE TO LEADERSHIP AND MANAGEMENT ON THE WARD

Jenny Thomas MA BSc (Hons) PGCHE RGN

Senior Lecturer, London South Bank University,
London, UK

SECOND EDITION

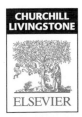

CHURCHILL
LIVINGSTONE

ELSEVIER

EDINBURGH   LONDON   NEW YORK   OXFORD   PHILADELPHIA
ST LOUIS   SYDNEY   TORONTO   2013

CHURCHILL
LIVINGSTONE
ELSEVIER

First edition 2006
Second edition 2013
  Reprinted 2013, 2014

ISBN-13: 978-0-7020-4583-7

British Library Cataloguing in Publication Data
A catalogue record for this book is available from the British Library

Library of Congress Cataloging in Publication Data
A catalog record for this book is available from the Library of Congress

Note
Knowledge and best practice in this field are constantly changing. As new research and experience broaden our knowledge, changes in practice, treatment and drug therapy may become necessary or appropriate. Readers are advised to check the most current information provided (i) on procedures featured or (ii) by the manufacturer of each product to be administered, to verify the recommended dose or formula, the method and duration of administration, and contraindications. It is the responsibility of the practitioner, relying on their own experience and knowledge of the patient, to make diagnoses, to determine dosages and the best treatment for each individual patient, and to take all appropriate safety precautions. To the fullest extent of the law, neither the Publisher nor the Author assumes any liability for any injury and/or damage to persons or property arising out of or related to any use of the material contained in this book.

ELSEVIER your source for books, journals and multimedia in the health sciences

www.elsevierhealth.com

Working together to grow
libraries in developing countries

www.elsevier.com | www.bookaid.org | www.sabre.org

ELSEVIER   BOOK AID International   Sabre Foundation

The
Publisher's
policy is to use
paper manufactured
from sustainable forests

Printed in China

A NURSE'S
SURVIVAL GUIDE TO
LEADERSHIP AND
MANAGEMENT
ON THE WARD

For Elsevier:
Content Strategist: Mairi McCubbin
Senior Content Development Specialist: Ailsa Laing
Senior Project Manager: Sukanthi Sukumar
Designer: Miles Hitchen

Contents

Preface

The role of ward manager is so important yet so overlooked in today's health care system. Unfortunately, the role has become so huge that some are struggling to keep up with the day-to-day demands of running shifts and completing all the paperwork, leaving little time or energy left to lead nursing. There are few specific training programmes, which means that learning often takes place through trial and error. This is not the most effective way to build up the skills and confidence required to lead. In addition, it is a rather isolated role at a time when support is probably most needed in your career.

I spent many years as a ward manager, yet it was not until I reached senior manager/deputy director level that I finally found out the things I should have known back then. No one told me how to run a budget; I just started receiving budget statements each month. No one told me how to investigate and write a complaint response; I simply assumed that what I did was right because no one told me otherwise. In fact, I still didn't know the proper procedure until I spent a year afterwards working in a complaints department. I attended numerous management courses and learned about various management theories and models, but few gave specific information on how to do things in real life. I still picked up most of my job through experience – not ideal.

I now provide teaching programmes, facilitate workshops and support groups for ward managers and matrons, and have been asked many times which book I got my information from. But there was no book. Most of the content in this book is taken from nearly 30 years of personal experience and observations. I gained a lot of this information from all the jobs I have had in health care *since* being a ward manager.

This book differs from other management and leadership books in that it is a practical guide; it is not an academic book. It is written in everyday language, specifically avoiding management jargon and academic theories. It also includes tips on how to cut through red tape and bureaucracy and put the patient first.

This is basically a 'how-to' book. When you need to look up how to do something, the last thing you need to do is wade through lots of academic theory. You will find this book helpful whether you are planning to be a ward manager, have recently taken on the role or even if you have many years of experience in the role. Matrons will also find it a useful guide for teaching and developing their teams. Although the book is aimed specifically at ward managers, it can be applied to clinical managers of any setting including A&E, ICU and outpatients.

This second edition has been updated to reflect the current health care environment which has changed markedly over the past few years. There is a greater focus on achieving set performance/quality indicators with the added pressure of delivering a more effective service for less cost. There are tips throughout the book on dealing with these pressures while ensuring that care remains patient centred and you and your staff do not burn yourselves out trying to deliver the impossible.

The increased focus on learning from our mistakes and being open about them has been taken into account with the addition of a new chapter which takes you through the current guidance on 'Improving quality and safety'.

The first eight chapters concentrate on the basic skills required for the ward manager's role. The next few chapters (9–12) give information on how to be more effective in your role. And finally, Chapters 13–16 discuss common problems for ward managers, suggested solutions and where to go for the most appropriate advice.

This book can be easily read through from cover to cover. It contains useful action points at the end of each chapter, which you may wish to use to inform your personal development plan. It can also be used as a handy reference book in times of need. You can look up quickly how to deal with an allegation of bullying, for example, or how to calculate your team's study leave allowance.

Although the content of the book is mainly based in the context of the NHS, it is also relevant for those working in private health care. Most private health care companies base their policies and procedures on at least those required within the NHS sector. In England, all private providers have been required to register with the Care Quality Commission since April 2011, and are therefore subject to the same care standard regulations as NHS organisations.

I hope you enjoy reading this book and that it provides you with the support and practical information you need to do the job effectively, and to keep yourself sane in what must be one of the most difficult and demanding jobs within health care.

London 2011   Jenny Thomas

ABOUT THE AUTHOR

Jenny Thomas has worked in health care for nearly 30 years including several years as a ward manager, matron/senior nurse and deputy director of nursing. She has considerable experience in supporting and developing ward managers and matrons and still works with these groups as a senior lecturer at London South Bank University. She holds academic and professional qualifications in nursing, management and education.

Acknowledgements

A big thank you to my esteemed colleague Dr Louise Terry (Reader in Law and Ethics) for her valuable and necessary contributions to Chapter 1.

I am also grateful to all the ward managers, sisters and charge nurses who have taken part in my courses over the years sharing their stories and stimulating many of my ideas for the book and this second edition.

And lastly, I must mention my work colleagues (you know who you are) who have been so patient with me, reading through my chapters and gently correcting my grammar, copious colloquialisms and other sundry matters.

Abbreviations

AOB	any other business
BNF	British National Formulary
CNO	Chief Nursing Officer
CNST	Clinical Negligence Scheme for Trusts
CPR	cardiopulmonary resuscitation
CRB	Criminal Records Bureau
ECG	electrocardiogram
FAQs	frequently asked questions
HCA	health care assistant
HDU	high-dependency unit
HR	human resources
ITU	intensive treatment unit
JCNC	Joint Consultative and Negotiating Committee
JSSC	Joint Staff Side Committee
KSF	knowledge and skills framework
LHB	local health board
MRSA	methicillin-resistant *Staphylococcus aureus*
NMC	Nursing and Midwifery Council
NSF	national service framework
OH	occupational health
PALS	patient advice and liaison services
RCA	root cause analysis
RCN	Royal College of Nursing
WTE	whole time equivalent

BE CLEAR ABOUT THE ROLE OF THE WARD MANAGER

When you become a nurse manager your responsibilities change. Most of your education and experience to date will have been focused on clinical practice, but the manager's role requires a very different set of skills. You are required to manage a team of staff with a set budget and are responsible for maintaining an environment in which people can work well.

Being a good nurse does not necessarily mean that you are naturally a good nurse manager. The two roles are very distinct. As a nurse, you are responsible for providing patients with a high standard of care. As a nurse manager, you are responsible for providing patients with a high standard of care *through others*. It takes time and experience to learn the art of being a good manager. Clarifying exactly what is expected of you in your role is the first major step.

BE CLEAR ABOUT WHAT 24-HOUR RESPONSIBILITY MEANS

Ward managers carry 24-hour responsibility for the ward. This means you are required to ensure that systems and processes are in place for patients to receive a high standard of care from your team, day and night, irrespective of whether you are there or not. It also means that you could be liable for poor patient care when you are not there if it is evident that you did not do everything to ensure that those systems and processes were in place. This includes:

- the appropriate development and support of your staff
- appropriate policies, guidelines and standards
- adequate rosters
- sufficient risk management activities.

The individual nurses in your team are registered professionals and therefore responsible and accountable for their own actions or inactions, under the terms of their registration. However, as their manager, you may be liable if you do not provide the right working conditions for your team to provide good care.

BEING CALLED AT HOME IS UNACCEPTABLE

The term '24-hour responsibility' does not mean that you should be accessible out-of-hours. It is a common misconception that the ward manager should be available at all times. There have been instances when on-call or site managers have called ward managers at home or on their mobile phones to sort out issues. You do not receive any payment for this, so it is unwise to encourage it. Home distractions or tiredness could also impair your response.

It is different if you have not done your job properly. For example, if some staff do not turn up for work on your ward one day and it is not clear on the roster who should be working that shift, then that is your responsibility. It means that you did not ensure adequate cover in your absence, and therefore need to be contacted to clarify matters. However, if members of your staff call in sick when you are not there, leaving shifts uncovered, it is the responsibility of the shift leader, matron or site manager to deal with the problem.

It is also not appropriate for members of your own team to be calling you at home. Your role is to enable them to make their own decisions and not to have to call you out-of-hours for advice. It is the responsibility of both you and your organisation to ensure that other senior managers are there to turn to for advice and support in emergencies when you are not there. This is usually the matron during office hours and some sort of on-call or site manager out-of-hours. If there is no such system properly in place, you could be liable for failing to address this omission.

MINIMISING RISK

Having 24-hour responsibility for your ward means you must minimise the risk of anything untoward happening in your absence by ensuring that:

- the appropriate health and safety procedures are in place
- the appropriate resources are available, including staff
- all members of your team have full access and have been made aware of all the appropriate policies and guidelines to inform them of the standards expected
- all members of your team have had appropriate induction and ongoing development to ensure they are competent in their role.

YOUR PROFESSIONAL AND MANAGERIAL ACCOUNTABILITY

The Nursing and Midwifery Council (NMC) does not offer any specific guidance on the accountability of nurse managers. However, it does include the aspect of being accountable for how and when to delegate. The NMC code (NMC 2008) requires that, when delegating, you must:

- establish that anyone to whom you delegate is able to carry out your instructions
- confirm that the outcome of any delegated task meets required standards
- make sure that everyone you are responsible for is supervised and supported.

In 2002, one of the reasons for removing a matron from the register was cited as placing 'unreasonable demands on staff'. A unit manager was also removed for 'failing to take appropriate action when a patient was assaulted by a member of staff'. In other words, as a manager who is also an NMC registrant, you are failing to uphold the code if you do not put the interests of the patients first in any managerial decisions that you make. This is also made clear in the code of conduct for NHS managers (Department of Health 2002) which states that 'the care and safety of patients' should be your first concern and you must 'act to protect them from risk'.

RAISING CONCERNS

If you are working under extreme pressure or there are staffing shortages out of your control, you must report it to the appropriate senior manager and be able to demonstrate that you have made every effort to remedy the situation. Again, this is made clear in the NMC code which also adds that 'you must report your concerns in writing if problems in the environment of care are putting people at risk' (NMC 2008).

You should also be alert to pressures being felt by your staff, since overworked staff may act inappropriately. In 2011, the NMC found 'basically a good nurse' with 'no evidence of general incompetence' who was 'dedicated to a career in nursing' guilty of misconduct when she failed to summon assistance or commence resuscitation on a pulseless patient and completed the patient's fluid charts retrospectively. In another case, the High Court held that the NMC had been unduly lenient in not finding unfitness to practise on the part of a midwife who failed to provide support to a junior colleague undergoing preceptorship and subsequently spoke in a bullying and intimidatory manner towards the person who had reported her. It is important to raise concerns over staff pressures rather than raise your voice to staff.

The NMC has produced clear guidelines for raising concerns to help all nurses and midwives (NMC 2010) and the Royal College of Nursing (RCN) in Northern Ireland has produced some good guidelines which are particularly relevant for ward managers and shift nurses-in-charge (RCN 2010). These guidelines also detail what you should include when raising your concerns in writing, such as:

- evidencing your concerns
- being specific
- identifying actions that you have already taken
- being precise about exactly what is needed to remedy the situation
- asking for an acknowledgement of your concern.

If your line manager fails to address your concern, then you should raise it with your organisation's designated person. Every organisation is required to have a designated person with specific training and responsibility for dealing with escalated concerns. For nurses and midwives, it's usually (but not always) the director of nursing. Only ever consider taking your concerns further (e.g. regulatory organisation, MP or media) once you have exhausted these routes within your own organisation, and never do so until you have sought advice from the NMC, RCN or other trade union. Public Concern at Work is an independent charity which also offers free advice in such situations (www.pcaw.co.uk).

BE CLEAR ABOUT WHAT MAKES A GOOD LEADER

OK, so your job title is a 'manager'. This does not automatically make you a good leader. Your job is to manage staff and resources to ensure that patients on your ward receive a good standard of care. If you lead well, your job as a manager will be made far easier. The job of a manager is to ensure people get things done, whereas a leader guides and inspires people and asks them how we can get things done. A good leader also enables their team to question whether the things need doing in the first place.

There are various leadership models being promoted within health care. The main ones at the moment are transformational and shared or distributed leadership.

TRANSFORMATIONAL LEADERSHIP

Transformational leadership is about influencing others to do things. The transformational leader is charismatic and inspirational. They are more considerate towards individuals. They stimulate people to be more creative and to challenge the system if necessary. The opposite of transformational is transactional. Transactional leadership applies to the older managerial style of setting tasks, giving rewards to those who achieve them and 'punishing' those who do not.

It is debatable as to whether transformational leadership is the model that is actually being used throughout practice at the moment, or whether it is entirely appropriate, since the current emphasis on meeting performance indicators can be viewed as largely transactional. However, a transformational leader will not only ask their team how indicators can be met, they will also question them and look at alternative solutions if they are detrimental to the overall patient care. So even in a transactional organisation, you can be transformational in your approach.

To become more transformational in your style, it would be worth considering the five practices of good leadership based on 30 years of research by Kouzes and Posner (2011). These are to:

- inspire a shared vision
- model the way
- challenge the process
- encourage the heart
- enable others to act.

Inspire a shared vision. Get the team together and ask them about where they all want to be in the future, or more realistically in a year's time. Facilitate them to set specific objectives together that they are all willing to work towards.

Model the way. Set an example about the standards you want your team to achieve and give them regular individual feedback about their progress. Show them how to cut through the bureaucracy.

Challenge the process. Continually question and look for ways of improving care in your ward. Encourage your staff to question decisions made by others (including other health professionals), by having the appropriate knowledge, confidence and support in order to do so.

Encourage the heart. Maintain morale by being continually optimistic and encouraging your staff in their work. Praise them when they do things well.

Enable others to act. Enable your staff to make important decisions and take risks by investing in their development and support.

SHARED LEADERSHIP

The inquiries into Maidstone and Tunbridge Wells (outbreaks of *Clostridium difficile*) and Mid-Staffordshire (higher than average mortality rates) clearly showed failures in leadership, not only at the top of these organisations but throughout the organisations, as clinicians felt powerless to do anything. Scandals such as these have highlighted the need for all clinicians to be leaders, and develop the skills to take action in such situations. Shared leadership is about all health care workers being able to see what needs doing or what needs to change and having the skills to work with others in order to do it. Clinicians should develop the leadership skills to work in partnership with experienced non-clinical managers and vice-versa.

THE NHS LEADERSHIP FRAMEWORK

The NHS Leadership Framework is based on shared leadership, although it still contains elements of transformational style as well as general management competences (National Leadership Council (NLC) 2011). It has five core domains based on:

- demonstrating personal qualities
- working with others
- managing services
- improving services
- setting direction.

For more senior managers, such as those at board level, there are further domains which concentrate on leadership at a more strategic level:

- creating a vision
- delivering the strategy.

Staff can progress through various stages. Members of your team should be encouraged to develop competences at stage 1, which is within their own team. This stage is about developing good working relationships with their co-workers, and developing the skills to both recognise problems and work with others to solve them. The next stages, 2, 3, and 4, build on the skills of people in managerial positions, including that of ward manager, to build on the skills entailed in working across teams, the organisation and the whole health care system.

Various development programmes are available for ward managers through the NLC (www.nhsleadership.org.uk), King's Fund (www.kingsfund.org.uk/leadership) and RCN (www.rcn.org.uk/development/practice/leadership). It's worthwhile accessing one of these types of programmes which are focused on clinical leadership rather than general management.

MAKE SURE YOUR DECISIONS ARE INFORMED ONES

If you make decisions that affect your staff or patients based on the advice of one person alone, you cannot blame them if your decision was the wrong one. If there is a serious incident, for example, and you take a course of action that your manager advised, you may remain fully responsible for the outcome of that decision. So get advice from others as well before you make that decision. Make sure all your decisions are informed ones.

YOUR LINE MANAGER

Try not to rely on your line manager as your only source of advice. They are not necessarily the best people to guide you in your work. Not all line managers have been ward managers and know what the role entails. And of those who have had experience, how can you be sure that their experience is any better than yours and that they are giving you the right advice?

Sometimes nurses rely too heavily on the next person above them within the hierarchical system. This can be a mistake as, nowadays, being more senior does not necessarily mean that you have more relevant experience. That's not to say you should ignore the advice and guidance of your line manager. Indeed, there are some very good and experienced matrons and service managers. However, it is always advisable to seek guidance from a variety of sources so that you can make an informed choice.

YOUR MENTOR

As a ward manager, you should find yourself a mentor; preferably someone several ranks higher than you. If possible, try and get one of the board directors to be your mentor. Most board or assistant board directors are keen to mentor someone from the clinical setting within their own organisation. A senior manager from another hospital or even a non-health care setting would be advantageous, particularly in helping you with human resource (HR) issues (see Ch. 10 for further information on mentorship in management).

YOUR CLINICAL SUPERVISOR

It would also be wise to have a clinical supervisor. You need to have someone who is more expert than you in your specialist area to help you reflect and learn from your clinical practice. This could be a nurse specialist, consultant doctor/nurse or another more experienced ward manager (see Ch.5 for further information on clinical supervision).

THE HR DEPARTMENT

Do not rely solely on your line manager or colleagues for advice regarding personnel issues. You may be able to benefit from their experience with similar issues but make sure you also consult with HR before making any decisions. If you have problems with your staff, such as inappropriate behaviour, sickness/absence problems or incompetence, your HR department will be able to provide the most up-to-date information with which you can then make the most appropriate decision.

Make sure you build up the appropriate networks before any problem arises. You should be meeting with your HR advisor on a monthly basis to build up a good working relationship. This will help enormously in times of crisis.

THE FINANCE DEPARTMENT

If you are going to make any changes at all which may involve extra staff or resources, always consult with your finance advisor first. It is their job to calculate the cost of any changes and to advise you what the best course of action is in terms of resources. They can help you become involved in the business planning process for your directorate and you will become far more knowledgeable and effective in accessing appropriate resources. As with HR, you should be meeting with your finance advisor on a monthly basis.

OTHER WARD MANAGERS

Another incredibly valuable resource often ignored by many ward managers and deputy ward managers is that of other more experienced ward managers. Why do so many ward managers work alone without searching out support from their more experienced peers? If you don't have some sort of group where ward managers get together to share experiences, guide and support each other, it would be a good idea to develop one yourself (see p. 177).

CLARIFY YOUR OBJECTIVES

Within 3 months of starting your job, you should have a formal performance review with your manager to clarify your objectives. If your manager does not arrange this automatically, take the lead and make it happen. You should have 3 months first to settle in and identify what needs doing and any further skills that you require to meet those needs.

Your manager will also have specific objectives that you are required to fulfil. These usually relate to quality indicators such as the number of complaints, pressure ulcers or infection rates. You may have your own objective such as implementing team nursing, self-rostering or increasing staffing levels. The aim of the performance review is to clarify your objectives together. At your first meeting, you should:

- review where you are now
- agree your objectives and how these will be achieved
- identify the skills you require to achieve the objectives.

A performance review at this stage will ensure that you both agree what your priorities are. There will always be more demands than you can meet. You have to agree with your manager which tasks are more important. You may see that all the patient information leaflets need updating, for example, but if you do not have enough staff to fulfil your minimum staffing requirements, your priority will be to recruit more staff over the next 6 months. Having this set out formally will stop you taking on lots of extra tasks. It will stop you working in a different direction to that of your manager.

You should also discuss and understand your line manager's own objectives. Part of your role is to assist your manager in achieving their organisational objectives. You should be working together towards the same goals. The performance review process helps to ensure this happens.

PREVENT WORK OVERLOAD

Every time you find that there are more things that need to be changed or improved, do not go ahead and attempt to add them to your workload. Concentrate on your objectives. If you feel that your long-term priorities need to change, arrange a meeting with your manager to discuss and, if necessary, change your agreed objectives.

Review your progress towards your objectives with your manager regularly. Priorities change frequently and your objectives should reflect these changes. In addition, frequent reviews help you and your manager understand and appreciate your role and responsibilities.

FIND OUT WHAT YOU NEED TO KNOW

One problem with being a ward manager is how do you know what you need to know? How do you know that you are doing the job right? This is especially pertinent if your manager has never been a ward manager, has only a few years' experience or their experience in the role is limited to one ward only.

Having a wider network is pivotal to ensuring you have access to a wider source of knowledge. Take time to set up good links with other ward managers and departments such as HR, finance and facilities. Assess where you are now. You can use your job description to guide you, or the knowledge and skills framework (KSF) and build on that assessment. Alternatively, assess yourself using the questionnaire provided in Appendix 1.1. This may help you to identify what you need to know.

360-DEGREE FEEDBACK

Another way of assessing where you are now is to undertake a 360-degree review. This is becoming an increasingly popular method of gaining feedback from others. It involves filling in a questionnaire assessing yourself against certain criteria and asking your managers, your team and your peers to also fill in the same questionnaire about you and your performance.

You can have a formal 360-degree review using the NHS Clinical Leadership Competency Framework (NLC 2011), in which the questionnaires are sent out on your behalf and all the information gathered into a report for you. You can work through this with a trained facilitator who will help you learn from the report in terms of understanding your strengths and helping you to determine areas that you would like to improve.

UNDERSTAND YOUR LEGAL RESPONSIBILITIES

Addressing adverse incidents and accusations of negligence costs the NHS a lot of time and money and causes managers and staff immense anxiety. Legal actions can take years to resolve, meaning years of stress. You may have to defend your actions or inactions in court. You may find yourself named repeatedly as the person responsible in a coroner's verdict, which is a public document, as was one nurse who gave a patient ten times the correct dose of medication, leading to the patient's death in 2009.

Most nurses are aware of their legal and professional liability for their individual practice. Patients are owed a duty of care by the hospital and by the individual staff delivering care. The question then is whether that care has been delivered negligently. Ask yourself: What would a reasonable manager do in this situation? What guidelines, protocols or evidence can you produce in justification?

TENSIONS BETWEEN ROLES OF NURSE AND MANAGER

As ward manager, you will be liable as a nurse for your personal nursing actions and as a manager you will be liable for your managerial actions. Tensions can arise between the two roles. For instance, pressure on beds might mean early discharge of a patient. As a nurse you may recognise that discharge is not in the patient's best interests but as a manager you are under pressure to maintain the service and know that the patient being admitted is in greater need of the bed. If the patient who is discharged early suffers harm, whether you were negligent in some way or not might depend upon whether evidence can be shown that the discharge was in accordance with ward or hospital guidelines and the proper procedures were followed. In 2010, a teenager died after having become 'lost' in a hospital following various moves by the bed manager to inappropriate wards rather than intensive care. The patient was finally moved to an intensive care unit when a junior doctor finally noticed her 'effectively moribund' condition.

You have a responsibility to address factors that might result in poor patient care. These factors may include:

● incompetent or inexperienced staff, whether members of your team or the wider interdisciplinary team
● poor English (both spoken and written)
● poor skill mixes
● lack of permanent staff
● inadequate resources
● unethical or illegal practice
● bullying.

If you don't address these factors, in law you may be seen as adopting these bad practices and so become liable yourself.

STAFFING SHORTAGES

Sometimes it is impossible to get sufficient qualified staff for a shift. This may be an ongoing problem on your ward. Ensure a proper record is made, submit the appropriate incident form and work with senior managers to find ways to address the problem. In addition to this, you *must* make sure that you make changes to the workload to maintain patient safety. If a patient inadvertently suffers harm in that situation, you should be able to show that as a reasonable, responsible ward manager you met your duty of care.

In 2008, the court heard a case where a neonatal intensive care nurse had two babies to care for where 'ideally any such nurse should be tasked to care for just one baby but the exigencies of the NHS regime made caring for two babies practically inevitable'. There was no evidence that she checked the baby's blood pressure during the night and the baby's deterioration was not identified in a timely manner. The court also noted that the failures to react came towards the end of the shift, 'a very busy time as preparations are made for handover'. It seems that the baby's care was being shared with the ward sister who was busy doing patient care, records and handover while the baby's named nurse was elsewhere.

SENDING STAFF TO OTHER WARDS

You may be asked to send a member of your team to help on an understaffed ward. You need to consider whether this will put any of your patients at risk. Your duty is towards your own patients. You may also find that members of your staff refuse to go when asked. Listen to the reasons they give, and ensure you are not asking them to undertake any responsibility for which they do not have the knowledge or skills. It is better to find out why they refuse to go and identify what would help the situation, such as an agreement with the requesting ward manager on what the member of staff can or cannot do.

VICARIOUS LIABILITY

Usually, if fault is established, the employing hospital is vicariously liable for the actions of their employees, which means that they pay the compensation to the victim. However, sometimes they can claim all or some of that compensation back from the employee, which happened in the case of Trustees of London Clinic v Michael Alan Edgar (2001) when a surgeon was held partially liable for nurses' postoperative inactions following a poor handover. The hospital settled out of court but then recovered £30000 from the surgeon.

Ensure that you have insurance through union membership. The employing hospital might also be fined so 'those in management roles' ensure that 'staff recognise the importance of being up to the mark.' A hospital was fined in 2008 under the Medicines Act 1968 when the volumes of glucose and vaminolact for a baby's feed were entered wrongly into a machine and the baby died of massive glucose overload. The Court of Appeal noted that the fine was equivalent to the annual salaries of two and a half nurses.

EXPANDED ROLES

Nurses are constantly expanding their roles. Your role as manager is to ensure that changes in practice are properly implemented. One trust agreed that midwives could top up epidurals if trained and assessed as competent by anaesthetists. Over the years, without the trust realising, this slid into midwives showing other midwives without any formal assessment of competency. An error was made resulting in injury to a patient. It was held that the midwife was acting outside her scope of practice. Furthermore, the trust could have said that she was 'on a frolic of her own' and expected her to pay compensation to the patient out of her own resources.

DUTY TO REPORT CONCERNS REGARDING A STRATEGIC DECISION

Occasionally, a hospital is held to have primary liability. In other words, the hospital's own negligence is the cause of harm. In one case, a hospital decided to employ only one obstetrician at night even though maternity services were on two sites. Lack of timely care meant a twin boy was left brain-damaged even though all the staff present had acted entirely professionally and competently. If a strategic decision by your hospital could put patients at risk, you have a professional duty to report concerns.

DUTY TO REPORT CAUSES FOR CONCERN REGARDING VULNERABLE ADULTS

A vulnerable adult is defined as anyone aged 18 years or over 'who is or may be in need of community care services by reason of mental or other disability, age or illness; and who is or may be unable to take care of him or herself, or unable to protect him or herself against significant harm exploitation' (Department of Health 2000). All such adults that are admitted to your area should be identified and have an appropriate individualised care plan which takes account of their individual needs and circumstances, with the involvement of the person's carer/family.

Vulnerable adults who lack capacity to make their own decisions may need to be protected from harm by measures such as locking ward doors so people with dementia cannot wander off. Since April 2009, the Mental Capacity Act 2005 Deprivation of Liberty Safeguards (MCA DOLS) requires all hospitals and care homes to carry out an assessment in such cases to decide whether the care or treatment is being given in a lawful manner. If a person with an MCA DOLS authorisation is transferred from a care home to a hospital and the ward needs to continue to restrict that person's liberty, a fresh MCA DOLS assessment must be carried out.

You must ensure that your team are alert to possible cases of abuse when dealing with vulnerable adults. This includes all patients who are dependent due to chronic or acute illness, plus those who:

- are elderly and frail
- suffer from mental illness
- have learning disability
- have a physical or sensory disability
- suffer from severe physical illness
- suffer with substance misuse.

Abuse can mean anything from physical, psychological or sexual abuse to actual neglect, discrimination or even financial/material abuse. Ward managers need to be alert to signs of abuse in their patients and also in vulnerable family members, both adults and children. The Office of the Public Guardian (2008) Safeguarding Vulnerable Adults policy includes a comprehensive list of possible indicators of abuse and causal factors (www.publicguardian.gov.uk). If any of your team suspects any type of abuse, they must report it to you, and you must report it promptly to your line manager and follow your local policy for safeguarding vulnerable adults. Remember that staff should record the comments using exactly the same words expressed by the vulnerable adult and should not question them concerning allegations or causes for concern.

There is a duty to refer anyone suspected to have caused harm or pose a risk of harm to a vulnerable adult to the ISA. If you have any concerns, you must raise them with your line manager and ensure they know how to make a referral to the ISA. From November 2010, it is illegal to employ people who are not registered with the Independent Safeguarding Authority (ISA) to work with vulnerable adults.

BE CLEAR ABOUT YOUR MATRON/LINE MANAGER'S ROLE

Your role is to support and develop your team. In turn, your manager's role is to support you and assist in your development. It is not your role to support your manager. If they need support, they should get this from their own line manager or mentor and not burden you with their problems. You have enough of your own. Don't take on your manager's problems as well. You may, however, need to encourage your manager to seek help. You may also have to report concerns about your manager as part of fulfilling your own legal and professional obligations. In any situation like this, always make sure you report your concerns in writing and seek support from elsewhere, such as your director or assistant director of nursing.

SHADOW YOUR MANAGER

It is a good idea to ensure you understand what your manager's role entails and the sort of problems they have to endure. One way to find out would be to spend some time shadowing your manager. Ask to accompany them to a couple of meetings so that you can see for yourself what the job is like and the pressures they are under.

'ACT UP' IN YOUR MANAGER'S ABSENCE

When you are more experienced, ask to 'act up' for your line manager to cover for annual leave. Make sure you get someone to 'act up' for you too. 'Acting up' in someone's absence does not mean carrying on doing your own job as well as covering theirs. 'Acting up' gives you a good insight into the other person's job. Make sure you have full responsibility for decision making and full access to the tools to do the job, e.g. their e-mail, post, agendas for meetings and what you are expected to contribute.

Make sure you have full handover before your manager goes on annual leave and give a full debrief on their return. You need to know what you did well and what you could have done better. It is the best way to learn from the experience. (Do the same for any members of staff who 'act up' in your absence.)

BUILD UP A GOOD WORKING RELATIONSHIP

Concentrate on building up a good working relationship with your manager. You need to understand their management style, including their preferred mode of communication. You also need to have a good insight into their priorities as well as their stresses and pressures. Part of your role is helping your manager to achieve organisational priorities. Make sure you work with them and not against them. If you do not agree with their decisions, say so. But make sure you put across your reasons and offer alternative solutions.

Be helpful but not adversarial. A good healthy working relationship is one in which either of you can challenge the other's decisions constructively without anyone feeling threatened in any way. Always show others that you and your manager work well together and communicate regularly. If people see any stresses and strains in your working relationship it will reduce their confidence in your management. They need to know that you are both in control.

You need to be able to decipher whether your manager is being reasonable. If you think your manager is not doing things right or is being a bit too bossy, how do you know if that's normal? How do you know that the reason you are not getting the right resources is because they are not putting your case forward in the business plan? The only way you will know is if you understand what their role is. You can also find out from your colleagues (other ward managers). If you maintain good communication with others, you can compare and contrast the role of their managers with yours.

Building up a close working relationship with your manager is so vital for success in your role that this book contains a whole chapter on the subject (see Ch. 12). Knowing and understanding their role is the first step to achieving this aim.

REMEMBER YOU ARE THE PATIENTS' OVERALL ADVOCATE

Advocacy is not just about ensuring the patient has the right information and support, it is about influencing a third party on behalf of patients (Teasdale 1998). Your role is to influence others to provide a high standard of care, to protect patients and speak up on their behalf. Yet it is still not unheard of for nurses and nurse managers to be referring patients and relatives to the Patient Advice and Liaison Service (PALS). This is a sad reflection on the role of the nurse as the patients' advocate.

PATIENTS NEED TO FEEL THAT THE MANAGER IS IN CONTROL

Patients and their relatives want someone to ensure that they get good care and that the level of care they get will not depend entirely on whichever individual they get to look after them. They want someone in charge who is able to make decisions and challenge poor practice (including government performance indicators if they are proving detrimental to the individual's care). They want someone to acknowledge when mistakes are made, ensure they are rectified and that something is done to ensure those mistakes don't happen again.

Patients are vulnerable and have no 'voice'. When a person becomes ill they are at the mercy of those assigned to care for them. Your role as the ward manager is to coordinate the health care team so the patient receives the best care.

It is not appropriate when a patient or relative makes a complaint to refer them to the complaints department or PALS or anyone else for that matter. This should only be done as a last resort. It is the ward manager's role to make sure the problem is sorted out in the first instance.

In order to act as your patients' advocate, you need to make time to be able to direct the care process. You cannot direct others if you are taking the same caseload as your staff. If you allocate yourself an equal number of patients as the rest of your staff, you are not managing. It indicates that you are not in control. Patients and relatives need to see that you are in control. They need reassurance that someone is:

● directing the team of nurses
● coordinating the doctors and other health care professionals
● challenging decisions that may not be appropriate
● ensuring that the focus on performance indicators is not detrimental to the quality of their care
● protecting them from individual incompetence.

But most of all they want to be reassured that someone is in charge of the ward and that someone has the time and experience to ensure that they are getting the right care. They want someone to be their overall advocate.

DON'T TAKE ON OTHER PEOPLE'S PRESSURES

The role of ward manager is probably one of the most highly pressured jobs within health care. You are responsible for the provision of patient care on your ward 24 hours a day, 7 days a week. What's more, most of the care is given through others. That is a huge responsibility. In other areas, senior managers are responsible for their area between the hours of 9 am and 5 pm, and they are rarely responsible for the actual care and treatment of vulnerable people. So don't take on their pressures too.

Many people working in health care seem to be always busy. Being busy all the time can mean they are not in control of their work. They have either taken too much on or are unable to prioritise their workload. They may not be competent or experienced in certain areas so their work takes twice as long as it would others. The work is controlling them. Bear this in mind when you are asked to take on a project or do a piece of work for someone else.

Don't take on other people's projects, unless it is something you wish to take on to learn and develop in your role. An example is the Essence of Care benchmarking project in England. Essentially, this is an audit tool to help you identify and make improvements to your area. Use it as such. Don't start becoming involved in endless discussions about other people's problems in the subgroups. Some nurses use these group meetings for general talking. Use a benchmarking group to gain ideas and share good practice. If the group is not doing that, either change the way it is being chaired or do not attend. Don't waste your time fulfilling other people's objectives for them.

BE WARY OF NON-CLINICAL MANAGERS

There are many non-clinical managers within health care. Certain jobs need to be undertaken by non-clinical managers in order to allow clinical managers the freedom to fulfil their clinical priorities. However, some take on projects that necessitate clinical involvement in order to achieve their outcomes. Without the clinical knowledge themselves, they will recruit those who do have the knowledge onto their working group. This is fine if you are expected to contribute your specialist opinion. It is not fine if you are being coerced into undertaking additional work to contribute to their project. If the work required does not fit into the objectives that you have previously agreed with your manager, then you should not be agreeing to do it. If you feel that the piece of work they have asked you to do is worth doing, you must then decide what current work you will give up in order to take on this project work. That is unless you do not have enough work to fill your time already!

The message is simple: don't waste time fulfilling others' goals at the expense of your own. That is not to say you should ignore the pressures that others have. Just don't make them yours.

DON'T ALLOW OTHER PEOPLE'S EMERGENCIES TO BECOME YOURS

Some managers will call meetings at a moment's notice and expect all to attend. Always clarify what the meeting is about first. Make an informed decision. If you have something more urgent to attend to, say so. Do not attend and then whinge. You made the choice.

When a senior manager calls for an urgent meeting, they may not realise that what you had planned is even more urgent. Non-clinical managers are not always aware of the importance of some of the things you do. Don't take on their pressures without making them aware of your own.

BALANCE YOUR CLINICAL WORK WITH ADMINISTRATIVE DUTIES

When you become a manager, you automatically take on a good deal more paperwork. This is one reason why you need to reduce your clinical time. A good ward manager will balance their clinical and administrative duties. If you do not manage this properly, you will end up either doing:

● too much clinical work: becoming part of the 'numbers' and catching up on the administrative work at the end of your shift or in your own time, or
● too much administrative work: becoming an office person, who becomes 'out-of-touch' with patient care or 'the real world'.

The key is to take control of these two aspects of your workload. As the ward manager, you should be allocating yourself the equivalent of 1 day per week for administrative work. Some call this their 'management' day. I have always thought this rather odd. Does this mean that they do not manage the rest of the time?

With any manager's role comes a fair bit of paperwork. You need to allocate yourself time away from the clinical area to go through it. Some argue that there is not enough money in the budget to do this. If this is the case, it is probably your fault for not having taken action to ensure it is in the budget. You therefore have two choices:

1. Work with your finance advisor to get this time added to your budget. This can be done either by putting it through as a business case or rearranging your staffing levels within the current year's budget.
2. Find some quiet time each day to spend 1 or 2 hours in the office. For example, you could work the mornings clinically and take 1–2 hours each afternoon in the office during the early–late shift overlap.

Do not take the work home. Taking work home with you because you do not have time during your working day is a bad habit. If you are working extra hours, either at work or at home, that is your decision, nobody else's. You have not been asked to do it and you are not paid for it. Therefore it is not being recognised by your employing organisation. Reprioritise your work to fit into the 37.5 hours per week that you are paid for (see Ch. 2).

REDUCE YOUR OWN PATIENT CASELOAD

The RCN produced a report on the role of the ward sister in 2009 which emphasises that all ward sisters should be supernumerary to shift numbers (RCN 2009). If you take on the same number of patients as each of your nurses on the shift, ask yourself:

1. What is the difference between what you are doing and the rest of the team?
2. Are you able to really support and manage your team?
3. Can you ensure constant observation of your staff and daily constructive feedback?
4. Can you maintain a good overview and control what is happening?

By taking on the same workload as your staff, you are in effect demeaning your role. You are working as a staff nurse but with the added responsibility of completing the paperwork. This is not managing at all. You are managing not to manage. It is a trap that many ward managers get into. They feel they are letting down their staff if they do not take on the same workload during the shift. In fact, they are letting down their staff by not taking care of aspects of management, such as ensuring the right budget and staffing levels.

You need to be able to give your staff more support. As the ward manager, you are more than just the nurse-in-charge of that shift. You need to take a longer-term view than just managing the shift. Your role is to ensure the right systems and processes are in place to enable your staff to carry out their duties to the best of their ability. You cannot do that if you are continuously in the numbers and just managing on a shift-by-shift basis.

You have to let go of some of the clinical work and balance it with the administrative side. It will help you ensure you are in control of your workload and therefore more effective.

BE AWARE OF THE IMPACT OF YOUR ROLE ON OTHERS

Your style of management not only affects the work of those in your team, it also affects other health professionals who have an input into the care of your patients. Try to ensure that the impact is always positive. Wards are often regarded as 'good' or 'bad' depending on who the ward manager is. Make sure people regard yours as one of the 'good' ones.

DOCTORS AND OTHER HEALTH CARE PROFESSIONALS

Make the effort to introduce yourself to all new staff, including doctors and medical students. You may find yourself working alongside them in a few years as consultants or GPs. Introduce a basic introduction package for all new doctors and other health care professionals. It doesn't take much to point out what the routine is, such as how the team nursing works, what is expected of them and what they can expect from you. You and your ward will soon get a good name and they will be more willing to help you if you have proved yourself to be helpful and welcoming in the initial stages.

The same goes for other health professionals such as physiotherapists, who are rarely based on one ward. Their patients are usually scattered all around the hospital. They soon get to know which ones are the nice wards and which are not. Don't let your ward be known as the one which everyone dreads entering.

STUDENT NURSES

The way you are perceived in your role is vital to the success of your ward and team. Think back to your student days and your ward placements. What influenced your opinion of the experience? Generally, it will have been the ward manager. Many students describe their placement experience in terms of what the ward manager was like. Your influence on others is immense. Be aware that whatever you do or say is under intense scrutiny and will be discussed among students back in the classroom. You cannot afford for any students to have 'a bad experience' on your ward. You want your ward to become the one where students are desperate to get a job once qualified.

In addition to this, role modelling of good patient care and good nursing practice is vital for student development. You must also ensure that students are not being used to fill ward shortages, so that they have proper opportunities to learn. However, there will be some students who, even with the best support, lack the necessary skills, so you must ensure that your mentors feel confident enough to fail them if necessary (see p. 73). Subsequent examination of his student placement packs showed that Colin Norris, a nurse who murdered several patients within a few months of qualifying, demonstrated behaviours which raised concerns over his suitability, but he was still passed by his mentors.

PATIENTS AND RELATIVES

Patients and relatives will also remember you. They are probably observing you more closely than anyone else. A good habit to get into is to ensure that you speak with every patient every day. While there are various initiatives in place, such as hourly rounding, to ensure all patients are seen by their nurse, it does make a difference if they see the ward manager each day. It will also help your staff if you can undertake one of their hourly rounds to enable them to pay attention to those patients who really need it.

Make a point of being available at visiting times too. Again, this will be a great support for your staff (enabling them to get on with their work) as well as dealing with the concerns of patients' relatives and carers

HOSPITAL MANAGEMENT

How you are perceived and carry out your role also has an impact on your line manager, your general manager and ultimately your chief executive and board of directors. You will leave yourself with no time to take part or challenge management decisions if you spend your time:

● taking on extra duties
● taking the same patient caseload as your staff each shift
● chasing up staff to cover for the day-to-day staffing shortages.

In order to make an impact on the hospital management, you have to involve yourself in the wider organisation and work together with other ward managers to ensure your voice is heard. If you choose to 'keep your head down' and concentrate on crisis management, you have only yourself to blame.

TAKE CONTROL

Take a step back, allow yourself some time to think and plan ahead. Try and be proactive rather than reactive. If you spend all your time managing details on a shift-by-shift level, someone else will make important decisions without your involvement because you are too busy. Ward managers also tend to work very much in isolation from their peers in equal positions. This makes their position weak within the overall organisation.

Don't always accept that there is nothing you can do and don't become a lone voice fighting for your corner in a huge organisation that doesn't have the time or the inclination to listen to you. Making yourself heard is a key managerial skill. It involves being able to prioritise your work better, knowing who's who, what makes your organisation tick and working closely with all the other ward managers. All these factors are included in this book, so your next action is to read through the rest of this book!

ACTION POINTS

- Assess your current role using the questionnaire provided in Appendix 1.1, and identify areas for improvement.
- Clarify your objectives with your manager within 3 months of starting your job and review them regularly.
- Explore the option of undertaking a clinical leadership or management course, if you have not already done so.
- Make sure there are specific written guidelines that outline the steps you and your staff should follow in the event of a shift being short staffed.
- 'Act up' for your manager to cover annual leave, as a learning opportunity.
- Be specific with others about what your role is and is not.
- Ensure there is an induction/information package for all newcomers to your ward, including doctors.
- Allocate the equivalent of 1 day per week to deal with the administration/paperwork.
- Reduce your patient caseload, see every patient each day and make yourself available at visiting times.
- Read the rest of this book!

References

Department of Health, 2000. No secrets: guidance on developing and implementing multi-agency policies and procedures to protect vulnerable adults from abuse. Department of Health, London. Online. Available: http://www.dh.gov.uk/en/ Publicationsandstatistics/Publications/PublicationsPolicyAndGuidance/DH_4008486 Jan 2012.

Department of Health, 2002. Code of conduct for NHS managers. Online. Available: http://www.dh.gov.uk/prod_consum_dh/groups/dh_digitalassets/@dh/@en/documents/ digitalasset/dh_4085904.pdf Jan 2012.

Kouzes, J.M., Posner, B.Z., 2011. The five practices of exemplary leadership, second ed. Pfeiffer, San Francisco.

National Leadership Council, 2011. The NHS Leadership Framework. Online. Available: http://www.nhsleadership.org.uk/framework-theframework.asp Jan 2012.

Nursing and Midwifery Council, 2008. The code: standards of conduct, performance and ethics for nurses and midwives. Online. Available: http://www.nmc-uk.org/Documents/Standards/ nmcTheCodeStandardsofConductPerformanceAndEthicsForNursesAndMidwives_Text Version.pdf.

Nursing and Midwifery Council, 2010. Raising and escalating concerns: guidance for nurses and midwives. Online. Available: http://www.nmc-uk.org/Documents/RaisingandEscalatingConcerns/Raising-and-escalating-concerns-guidance-A5.pdf Jan 2012.

Royal College of Nursing, 2009. Breaking down barriers, driving up standards: the role of the ward sister and charge nurse. Online. Available: http://www.rcn.org.uk/__data/assets/pdf_file/0010/230995/003312.pdf Jan 2012.

Royal College of Nursing, 2010. A practical guide to raising concerns for registered nurses. Online. Available: http://www.rcn.org.uk/__data/assets/pdf_file/0012/355899/Raising_concerns_final.pdf Jan 2012.

Teasdale, K., 1998. Advocacy in health care. Blackwell Science, Oxford.

Trustees of London Clinic v Michael Alan Edgar QBD, (19/4/2000, Hidden J) 2001. LTL.

APPENDIX 1.1

QUESTIONNAIRE TO HELP IDENTIFY DEVELOPMENT NEEDS FOR WARD MANAGERS

Leadership skills

- Does your team have a vision/goal of where you all want to be in a year's time?
- Do you have set objectives/actions that you have identified together to achieve that vision?
- Have you been able to change what is not right/working in your ward/department?
- Have you been able to change what is not right/working in your organisation?
- Have you had discussions with any of the board directors or general managers within the past 3 months about any issues in your ward/department?
- Are you actively involved in any trust-wide initiatives?
- Have you evaluated whether any recent changes in trust strategy could result in harm to your patients?
- Does your ward/department have a high profile within the trust because of high standards and/or quality indicators?

Education

- Are your staff fully trained and developed in all aspects of their work?
- Are you able to access all the educational resources you need for you and your staff?
- Do you know what percentage of your staffing budget is allocated for study?
- Do you plan your staff study leave a year in advance based on appraisal and keeping within the study leave limits?
- If yes to the above, do you involve your whole team in this planning?
- Are all your staff assessed against set clinical competences on a regular basis?
- Do all your staff have a local mentor/facilitator/coach to guide and support their development?
- Do you meet with your link tutor regularly and maintain close relations with the local university?
- Are all your staff up-to-date with their mandatory training?
- Are you making full use of the in-house and external development programmes to aid career progression of your staff?

Management of staff

- Have you had an appraisal/personal development plan agreed within the last year?
- Have all your staff been appraised within the past year?
- Do you know who your human resource advisor is?
- Do you meet with him/her regularly to discuss personnel issues (e.g. sickness/absence, staffing issues, recruitment)?

- Have you received training and development on staff management issues such as recruitment, policies and procedures, risk management, etc.?
- Do you have appropriate development programmes in place for your deputy ward sisters/charge nurses?

Management of budget

- Do you know what your budget is?
- Do you know what your budget is in terms of PAY and NON-PAY?
- Does your current budget reflect the skill mix required (as identified through a formal skill mix review)?
- Have you had any training and development on managing a budget?
- Do you contribute to the yearly business planning process?
- Do you meet with your finance advisor regularly?
- Are your staff all involved in managing the budget?
- Do you manage your team's annual leave throughout the year so that the ward does not have problems with 'meeting the numbers' in the January to March period?
- Do you have adequate resources for your ward in terms of staff and equipment?
- Do you know what services you have agreed to provide as part of your commissioned contracts?

Maintaining clinical standards

- Do you manage to see every patient on your ward every day?
- Are you happy that your staff are delivering care to a high standard every day?
- Would you be able to justify in court the way you allocate workloads and patients?
- Are your staff taking full responsibility for the care of their allocated patients?
- Do you have set standards/guidelines for all specialist procedures on your ward?
- Do you have a system within your ward of regularly reviewing themes from complaints, clinical incidents and local audits?
- Do you have a system of keeping your patients informed about the complaints themes and what you are doing about them?
- Are you confident that all your nurses are skilled enough to question inappropriate medical decisions?
- Do you have a plan of action for each serious incident and complaint within your ward/department?
- Do you have a clinical supervisor to constantly challenge you and enable you to keep up-to-date professionally?
- Have you and your team made any improvements to care within the past 6 months following patient feedback, results of complaints/incidents, audits or quality indicator monitoring?

Communication

- Do you meet with your team at least once each month?
- Do you open and deal with your e-mail on a daily basis?
- Do you appoint someone to 'act up' in your absence?

- Do you keep your matron fully informed of day-to-day operations and liaise on a regular basis?
- Are you fully aware of your responsibilities regarding the Freedom of Information Act and Data Protection Act?
- Does every member of your team have full access to a computer for e-mail, intranet and appropriate research to carry out their role effectively?
- Do you keep yourself and your team fully up-to-date about what is going on in the rest of your organisation?
- Do you ensure that your voice is heard at corporate level?
- Do you regularly get staff to shadow you?

Management of self

- Are you able to be a role model for your staff by working 37.5 hours per week, taking your meal/coffee breaks and still being effective?
- Do you plan your work at least a week in advance rather than just getting through everyday crises?
- Do you have a mentor who provides support as well as challenges you in your professional role?

Please note: This questionnaire is designed simply as an aid to stimulate thoughts and is not meant to be prescriptive or an exhaustive list of tasks that should be undertaken. You may find it helpful to identify those sections where there are mostly 'no' answers and think about what you can do to improve your skills in these areas.

MANAGE YOUR TIME

As mentioned in the previous chapter, putting in long hours at work does not necessarily mean you are good at your job. Being busy does not equate with being efficient and effective. It suggests that you are not in control. In order to manage your time more effectively, you need to have control over choosing what you do and how to do it. You also need to be able to choose what not to do. Spend your time accomplishing things, not just being busy. Invest time in planning, organising, rearranging, sorting and, most important of all, thinking.

This chapter focuses on how to manage your time more effectively and how to achieve a healthy work/life balance in your role.

DEFINE YOUR WORKLOAD

Most ward managers are employed to work 150 hours per month. It's worth taking some time to write down all the commitments you currently have in terms of hours per month, as indicated in Table 2.1. If the total hours add up to more than 150, it means that you do not have enough time to complete what is required. This indicates that in order to fulfil your workload, you are working more than 150 hours or not fulfilling your commitments. You may be:

- taking work home
- staying late regularly
- not getting things done.

Taking work home or staying late regularly?

If you have decided to take work home or stay on late regularly, this is not a sustainable option. You are not looking after yourself. You should be well rested, healthy and have a good work/life balance in order to be effective in your role. Plus, it is unpaid work. In other words, it is not recognised by your organisation or your manager. It is also not appreciated by the patients.

Not getting things done?

If the hours add up to more than 150 and you are not physically working all those hours, it means that some parts of your job are not getting done. You are probably finding that you are continually busy but don't seem to be getting on top of things. Things either get missed or get left undone.

Problems occur when you do not formally prioritise what gets done and what doesn't. It is often the case that clinical work takes less priority in order to get through the administrative work. That's a poor way to manage a ward. If you need to spend less time clinically, then plan it. Don't allow administrative work and meetings to take over and leave you feeling continually busy and overloaded. Both you and your staff will suffer.

PLAN AND PRIORITISE

Start by removing or reducing tasks in order to bring the total down to 150 hours. The first place to start is with the meetings. Do you really need to attend all those meetings? Choose the ones that are essential for the welfare of your patients and staff.

Do the same with any project work. Only keep the tasks that are essential. Essential work includes:

- doing the roster
- dealing with complaints

TABLE 2.1: Defining your workload in terms of hours per month

Description of task	*Total hours per month*
Meetings List the meetings you attend, including all one-to-one meetings (if weekly, multiply hours by 4, if quarterly divide hours by 3)	
1. e.g. Monthly sisters' meeting 2 h	2
2. e.g. Weekly ward team meeting 1 h	4
3.	
4.	
5.	
6.	
7.	
8.	
9.	
10.	
E-mails, voice-mail and post How many hours do you need per day for this? 30 mins - 1 hour am, 30 mins pm perhaps? (multiply this by 20 for the monthly figure)	
Investigating and writing responses to complaints (allow an average of 10 hours' work per complaint)	
Staffing issues (include appraisals, recruitment, etc.)	
Compiling the monthly roster	
Risk management and governance issues (average time spent on serious incident investigations, audits, pressure sore forms, etc.)	
Teaching (include preparation time)	
Own study/course commitments	
Regular admin/secretarial work (e.g. photocopying)	
Corporate or university work (e.g. 'block' recruitment, interviewing)	
Clinical (time spent on ward as part of clinical shift)	
Other (e.g. current project work)	
1.	
2.	
3.	
4.	
5.	
Total	

- dealing with incidents
- reading and dealing with e-mail each day
- managing and supporting your staff.

  Non-essential work includes:

- some project work
- some corporate work
- teaching externally to the ward.

Once you have worked out your commitments in terms of hours per month (using the prompts in Table 2.1), it is advisable to meet with your line manager to assist you in making the decisions required to reduce the non-clinical work if necessary.

The next step is to realistically identify how much time you have left to devote to clinical work. It may only be 70–80 hours per month. If that is the case, plan to split it into specific blocks of clinical time. This could be something like four half shifts per week. Devote that whole time to clinical work without going off to a meeting or into the office half way through. Let your staff see that you are in control of your work. If you need to keep interrupting your clinical shift to go off to meetings or into the office to catch up on paperwork, it shows that you are not in control of your workload. It is controlling you. Your staff will respect you far more if they see that you are in control of what you do.

ORGANISE YOUR OFFICE

Many ward managers have to share their office with others. Some offices double up as changing rooms, coffee rooms and in some cases they are the only place available to meet with relatives. If this is how it is with your office, try and designate at least one third of this room as your personal office space with your desk, computer and chair. Make sure all other chairs, coat hooks, beverages, etc. are kept on the other side of the room. You have the most important job on your ward and it is essential that you have some dedicated office space.

KEEP EVERYTHING YOU NEED TO DO ON ONE LIST

Write everything down on your list such as phone calls you need to make, messages to get back to people, reports to be written, project work, etc. All papers associated with your list should be filed away on your computer or in the filing cabinet. The list can run into three or four sheets of A4 paper but it doesn't matter, as long as everything is written down in one place. Keeping one list is simple but effective. It serves to greatly reduce your stress and worry by literally taking things off your mind and putting them down on paper. The basic concept is that you can stay on top and in control of all unfinished work, projects, reports and correspondence.

Get into the habit of noting down everything that requires an action and comes to you via post, e-mail, voice-mail, fax or phone on your central list of things to do. File e-mails and associated attachments on your computer if you need to keep them. Don't print them out. It's a waste of time and takes up unnecessary space on your desk or in your filing cabinet.

Set up an efficient filing system

If there are many files in your cabinet left by the previous post holder and you feel you may need to refer to them at some point, then use different types or colour of label for your own files so you can easily distinguish which are your own.

Never keep copies of documents if you can easily access them somewhere else. If you have a copy within your computer files, throw away the hard copy unless you will be referring to it often.

ENSURE THE OFFICE ENVIRONMENT IS IN GOOD ORDER

Keep your office space neat and tidy with no overflowing papers or post-it notes everywhere. Keep all stationery aids in a drawer, e.g. pens, stapler and paper clips. The only things directly on your desk should be your in-tray, computer screen plus keyboard and telephone. It is not always possible, but if you can, keep your printer on a different shelf/desk, preferably within easy reach of where you sit.

The location of your desk is very important. Your computer screen should be facing away from the window. Any glare from the daylight on your screen will cause strain on your eyes and headaches. Plants and photographs serve to make your office a nice place to spend your time but keep them away from your desk. Other personal items such as tea, handbags and umbrellas should be out of sight in a cupboard or drawer. Ensure you have adequate lighting. Order a desk light from your stationery budget. They are not expensive. It makes your office more comfortable and is better for reading. And one last very important tip is to always keep a store of printer cartridges. They tend to run out at the most inconvenient moment.

Having an organised office makes you far more efficient with your time. Less time and effort will be wasted looking for letters, documents and e-mails, and you will be far less likely to forget things.

CONTROL YOUR DIARY

When you are working a clinical shift, you plan what you are going to do after handover but it often changes due to patient need. You expect that to be the case. As clinicians we are used to continually altering our plans because looking after patients is unpredictable work. However, this approach doesn't work when dealing with the administrative side of your role. You cannot afford to spend your day reacting to events and constantly being interrupted. The time when you are not directly involved in patient care should be planned.

PRIORITISE YOUR 'TO-DO' LIST

The easiest way to plan your administrative work is to prioritise your list of things to do. Grade each task 1–3 in order of importance:

1. Urgent – needs to be done by today.
2. Important – if possible get done today, but can be left until tomorrow.
3. Can be left until next week.

It does not matter whether you have five or 50 tasks, it will make your life easier if you prioritise things. You can then concentrate on completing all those that are graded at priority 1.

It helps if you mark against each priority 1 task approximately how long that task will take. You can see at a glance which tasks will take just a few minutes, such as making a phone call. You can then concentrate on achieving those when you just have an hour or so in the office. Tasks such as reading or writing a report can be left for when you have a longer time slot.

DON'T KEEP REWRITING YOUR LIST

When you have completed a task, put a line through it rather than just putting a tick against it. This gives a greater sense of achievement. Administrative work does not give the rewards that you get from clinical work.

Don't rewrite it each day, as this would be too time consuming. Re-categorise the remaining tasks at the start of each day or at the end of each preceding day. Keep adding to the list depending on what happens during the day. Just rewrite the list when it starts becoming unreadable.

SET YOURSELF TIME LIMITS

Be realistic about what you can and can't do. Without limits, you end up being overstretched and working longer hours. Allocate a set time for each piece of work. Allow 1 hour to do an appraisal, for example, or 2 hours to prepare an important presentation. If the task is not finished by the end of the allocated time, set time for the next administration slot or submit the work as it is. It is no good striving for perfection all the time. Ask yourself, 'Will it do?' Aim to do things well enough. Doing them better than necessary is a waste of your valuable time.

TAKE YOUR BREAKS

Don't forget to schedule in your 30-minute lunch break. You are not paid for your lunch break, so don't work through it. Taking a proper 30-minute break will ensure you are refreshed and your batteries are recharged for the afternoon. You also need to set an example to your staff. If they know you take a proper lunch break they will follow suit. If you choose to eat a sandwich in the office while checking through e-mails, you will be seen as a poorly organised manager unable to manage your workload. It will make your staff feel guilty about taking their own lunch breaks.

PENCIL IN YOUR DIARY

Always use a pencil to write anything in your diary. Health care management can be very unpredictable. Meetings are frequently cancelled and rearranged at a later date. By using a pencil, you simply rub things out and save the page getting into an incomprehensible mess. Better still, use an electronic diary if you can.

BOOK ALL ANNUAL LEAVE IN ADVANCE

Book *all* your annual leave at the beginning of each financial year. Plan the time off for you and your family and friends. Many have lost annual leave due to poor planning. Something more important will always come up.

In order to keep yourself healthy and keep work in perspective, try to ensure you do not work more than 3 months without an annual leave break. It really is very important to be in control of your own time as well as your work time.

KEEP UP WITH YOUR E-MAILS

E-mail is now the main form of communication in health care management, so it's important to set aside time (at least 15–30 minutes) at the beginning and/or end of each day. Don't save them up for your 'admin' day. Also, try not to leave the ward every spare moment to catch up with your e-mails. It is not good time management but is an easy trap to fall into. When you are working clinically, you should concentrate on being there for your staff and patients.

DELEGATE YOUR E-MAILS TO SOMEONE ELSE IN YOUR ABSENCE

When you are on 'days off' or annual leave, delegate your e-mails to someone else to deal with. This could be your deputy ward manager, one of your staff nurses or even your ward clerk. It keeps your team informed when you are not there. It is a good development opportunity, particularly for junior sisters and charge nurses. Not only will they delete all the junk mail, read and answer the basic ones on your behalf, but also they will gain an excellent insight into your role and responsibilities. You must not give out your password, but you can enable certain named staff to have 'proxy access' to your e-mails. Ask your IT department to help you set this up if you have not already done so.

Confidentiality

If you are concerned about confidentiality, then perhaps you need to look at how you and your colleagues are using the e-mail service. You should never use your work e-mail account for private or personal e-mails. As a general rule, all your e-mails should come as no surprise if another member of your team gains access to them. Remember the golden rule: 'No e-mail is ever confidential'. Ensure all your team are aware of this. If you need to discuss confidential information, it should be done face-to-face or on the phone but never written in an e-mail.

FILE E-MAILS

Don't get into the habit of printing off e-mails or attached documents. Create various folders on your computer and file them as you would a piece of paper. Always use the organisation's shared drive to file e-mails away. This is the disk that is backed up each day centrally, so if your computer fails in some way you will not lose all your files. If you are saving your files on your personal computer (i.e. c:/drive), you risk losing them.

USING E-MAILS AS AN ESSENTIAL TIME MANAGEMENT TOOL

Always use e-mail in preference to the phone whenever you can. It saves a lot of time. Nowadays, if you phone, you rarely get the other person and end up leaving a voice-mail. They then call you and leave a voice-mail and this can go on for quite some time.

E-mails are an incredibly efficient way of working. They save much time but it does depend on the user. You should have a system with e-mails as you would with post. If you open post then leave it in your in-tray, it will get forgotten. The same is for e-mails. If, for example, you get an e-mail reminding you of a report you are supposed to be working on but haven't started, don't leave it in your in-box. Like the opened envelope left in your in-tray, it will get forgotten. Add the task within the e-mail to your 'to-do' list, then either delete or file the e-mail. And one more thing – don't allow e-mail to become another interruption to your working schedule: silence the beeper that sounds every time you receive an e-mail.

CUT INTERRUPTIONS

It is generally accepted that the ward manager or nurse-in-charge of the shift deals with all the queries and any tasks that are not directly patient related. When you are working clinically, you learn to deal with constant interruptions, but you cannot work like this when managing the paperwork side of your role. So when you plan time in your weekly diary for office work, you need to arrange cover on the ward. You cannot be in charge on the ward and work in the office at the same time.

WARD ROUNDS

Make sure you do a ward round every day. Most ward managers have some way of getting around to speak to all the patients and staff during the shift. This is often incorporated as part of the drug rounds, doctors' rounds, bedside handover or even a round of making beds. Making time to do this every day helps reduce those constant interruptions when you do eventually go into the office.

LET YOUR STAFF KNOW WHAT YOU ARE DOING IN THE OFFICE

Your staff must respect that you need uninterrupted time to deal with your administrative work. Let them know what you are doing. If you say you are short-listing candidates for interviews, compiling next month's roster or writing a business case for more equipment, they will understand why you need the time. If you say that you are going to the office 'to catch up on things', it doesn't sound quite so important. Health care professionals often see office work as unimportant compared to direct patient care, so make sure your staff are aware of exactly what you are doing rather than just calling it 'general paperwork'.

'OPEN DOOR' POLICIES DON'T WORK

Close your office door and tell people that you will accept interruptions for emergencies only. Leave a 'Do Not Disturb' notice outside, making sure that it is also dated with an indication of the time you need to remain undisturbed. This will lessen the risk of people popping in for general queries. They will be more likely to wait until the end-time given on the notice. When you are in the office:

1. If someone comes to your door asking 'Have you got a few minutes?', make a point of glancing at your clock or wristwatch before answering. Tell them exactly how much time you have or are prepared to give them. If you are in the middle of something, say so: 'I'm just finishing off a report; would you mind coming back at 4 o'clock when I can give you my full attention?', or 'I've got 5 minutes now if it is urgent, but if it can wait until 2 pm I'll have more time for you'.
2. Don't offer beverages to anyone who drops in unannounced. It indicates that you have plenty of time for tea and a chat.
3. Indicate the interruption is over by standing up. If they have not taken notice, show them to the door. Keep smiling throughout so the person does not feel awkward.
4. Don't make your office too welcoming. Do not have your desk facing the door. This encourages people to come in and interrupt you. Keep another chair appropriately placed in the room but well away from your desk. This deters visitors from staying too long.
5. Don't answer the phone while you are in the office. Leave it on voice-mail and allow 10 minutes at the end of your office session to go through your voice-mails. Make sure your voice-mail message indicates how you can be contacted in an emergency (preferably by pager).

DON'T WASTE TIME WITH UNNECESSARY READING

Reading can be very time consuming. In addition, keeping clinically up-to-date involves a lot of time not only reading but also searching for the relevant information. The NHS is particularly adept at producing massive documents, many of which you know you should read but will never really have the time. It is also difficult to know whether the document is important enough to be read or not. Learning the techniques of scanning and speed reading can be extremely helpful for all managers.

Scanning

Scanning helps you to get a feel for the content without reading it through. It saves you a lot of time and energy. With every new document, all you need to do is read:

- the title
- the introduction or executive summary
- the subheadings and the first and last sentence of each paragraph or section
- the conclusion.

Scanning can be applied to any sort of document. Try not to read any document or letter without scanning it first.

Speed reading

In addition, the average reading speed is around 250 words per minute. You can achieve double or quadruple this amount after 1 day's training. It is worth investing in a short course, which usually consists of 1–2 days. The basic technique is not to understand the actual words but to see the whole picture or concept of what is being said. You don't need to read each word to do this. The technique involves skimming across the page focusing on the main words in the sentence, not on the ones in between. That way, you can skim across paragraphs very quickly. It takes some practice to do this but can save a huge amount of time in the long term. Writing down key points from the document as you go also helps you to understand and remember what you have read.

JOURNAL ARTICLES

Don't keep piles of journals. You will rarely, if ever, refer to them. If you do need to refer to a journal article, you can access them online. Add a file labelled 'Current research' on your PC. If you see an article of interest in a journal, save it to your file and read later when you have time or print it off and leave it in the staff coffee room.

HOSPITAL NEWSLETTER AND INTERNAL BULLETINS

Leave any current information such as the hospital newsletter or internal bulletins on the coffee table in the staff room (even if it is the same room as your office). Renew them each week. It will help keep your staff up-to-date as well.

KEEP UP-TO-DATE WITH THE INTERNET

All ward managers should have full access to the Internet. Make full use of it. The World Wide Web is the quickest and easiest way of accessing information and

keeping you up-to-date. Make it a habit to access the NHS Web sites each month.
The following Web sites are useful for regular quick updates:

http://www.dh.gov.uk – The Department of Health's Web site for England
http://www.show.scot.nhs.uk – This is the official Web site of NHS Scotland.
http://www.wales.nhs.uk – The official Web site of NHS Wales.
http://www.dhsspsni.gov.uk/ – Department of Health, Social Services and Public
Safety in Northern Ireland.

Your hospital intranet site will keep you updated with what is going on in your
organisation.

As a ward manager, you need to keep abreast of the ongoing changes both
clinically and managerially. Being politically aware about what is going on in your
own organisation and in the NHS overall helps you to ensure your patients receive
the best from the system.

HANDLE MEETINGS EFFECTIVELY

Break the habit of going to meetings just because they are in your diary. Meetings
take up an awful lot of time in public service organisations. Some managers spend
so much time dashing from one meeting to the next that they leave themselves with
little time in which to do any work.

DON'T ALLOW YOUR CLINICAL EXPERTISE TO BE ABUSED

For each and every meeting, ask yourself 'Is it really necessary to attend?' Health
professionals are sometimes invited to meetings because the person in charge of the
project is not clinical and needs help and advice. As previously mentioned, this is
fine unless you are being delegated to undertake work for them. Beware of helping
others to achieve their goals/targets while falling behind on your own.

MEETINGS SHOULD NOT BE USED FOR DISSEMINATING INFORMATION

Meetings should be used for bringing together the right skills and experiences to be
able to make informed decisions and changes. A meeting is not required simply for
information-giving. There are far more efficient ways of giving information such as
e-mail, communication books and the hospital intranet. The purpose of meetings
should be to involve staff, not just to inform them.

AVOID BEING KEPT WAITING FOR APPOINTMENTS OR MEETINGS

If you have to meet with someone who is often late, ask them to come to you in
future so you avoid wasting your time waiting. Always take some reading with
you so when the person arrives after keeping you waiting, ask them to wait for

you while you finish what you are doing. If a regular meeting always starts late, get there on time and leave a note saying what time you left and where you can be contacted. This is a somewhat diplomatic way of getting your point across. It works particularly well with one-to-one meetings.

GETTING THE BEST FROM MEETINGS

Whether a meeting works or not depends entirely on the person running it. Few people have training in how to run a meeting. The following steps are important to get the best from meetings that you attend:

Step 1: Ensure the purpose has been specified
All regular meetings should have terms of reference (see Appendix 2.1). These make it clear what the meetings are for and the way in which they will be run. If any of the meetings you attend do not have written terms of reference, you should question why the meeting is taking place. Sometimes meetings are held when the distribution of a regular e-mail would suffice.

All one-to-one meetings should also have a specific purpose. 'To discuss the incident' is not specific enough. You need to have an outcome such as 'To identify what actions need to be taken following the incident'. Ensuring you have a specific objective stops you wasting valuable time discussing issues without achieving anything.

Step 2: Prepare
Notify the person running the meeting in advance if you have an agenda item and send them any supporting papers. Do not wait to raise it at the meeting as 'any other business' (AOB). AOB should be for urgent matters only. Read the minutes or action notes at least 1 day beforehand. This ensures that you are familiar with what happened last time and remember what you had agreed to do. It also gives you time to prepare your feedback about your actions if required. If you are not sure about any items on the agenda, ring up beforehand and ask. You cannot prepare or contribute if you do not understand what it is about.

Let people know if you cannot make it, will be late or have to leave before the end. It is considered rude to not turn up to a meeting without sending your apologies. Send an appropriate substitute if you can and, if you do, ensure that person is fully conversant with what the meeting is about, why they are there and that they are confident enough to speak up on your behalf.

For one-to-one meetings, send any items you wish to raise by e-mail in advance. This saves time and gives the other person time to prepare too.

Step 3: Know how to handle a poorly chaired meeting
This can be difficult to do without challenging or criticising the chair's competence. However, you can help to steer them in the right direction, with questions such as:

- Do you mind if we quickly run through the purpose of the meeting so I can be clear in my mind?
- Can you summarise that last point for us please?

- Last time we had the meeting, we took the current list of delayed discharges as a starting point. Perhaps it might be helpful if we took that approach again?

CHAIR MEETINGS EFFECTIVELY

The role of the person holding a meeting with a group of people is to act as the 'group facilitator'. This includes:

- enabling everyone to contribute or have their say
- ensuring the group comes to a decision or sets actions
- keeping to time
- utilising the best of the skills and experience in the room.

Before you chair any meeting, make sure you prepare beforehand:

1. *Familiarise yourself* with the agenda and previous minutes before the meeting.
2. *Sort out the room* to enable you to start on time and reduce interruptions, e.g. silence the phone, put a sign up outside the door and arrange the chairs.
3. *Send out the agenda and minutes* to reach individuals at least a week before the meeting if it involves people from other areas. This will not only remind them that the meeting is taking place but will also stimulate them to finish (or start!) the actions they agreed to undertake at the last meeting. Put these details up on your staff notice board or communication book if the meeting is for members of your team only.
4. *Start the meeting on time.* If someone comes in late, keep going. Acknowledge them with a nod only. Don't start again. If they sit down and ask where you are at, give a brief summary but don't hold everyone up by going through things all over again.
5. *Get everyone to quieten down and then welcome them.* Check that everyone has seen the agenda and minutes. Quickly run through the agenda to remind everyone what they are there for. Introduce any outside speakers and confirm their place on the agenda. Ask for any items under AOB.
6. *Keep the discussion on track.* If you find that people are becoming sidetracked, bring them back by saying something like 'This is a useful discussion, but we need to concentrate on the main issue. We can put that item on the agenda for a future meeting'.
7. *Control interruptions.* Your role is to ensure everyone has the opportunity to contribute. Deal with interruptions quickly or you will lose control of the meeting. Say something like 'Wait a minute, let X speak first, then we'll come back to your point …'.
8. *Observe everyone in the room.* Make sure that all have a chance to speak. Notice and act if someone is trying to speak but keeps being interrupted, or if someone looks bored or not in tune with what's going on. Notice if someone is aggressive, angry or upset. Say things like 'OK, maybe it's time to let someone else speak on this issue …' or 'What do you think, Wendy?' or 'Simon, you seem to be concerned about this, am I right?'

9. *Deal with conflict* by pointing out what is happening and saying something like 'Can we get back to the issue on the agenda please?' Usually that will nip things in the bud. If not, call for a break. Aggressive behaviour needs to be pointed out. Acknowledge the person's point of view but point out that this sort of discussion is not helpful and can be finished outside the meeting.

10. *Ensure everything runs to time.* All agendas should be timed. Preferably, the meeting should last an hour. No meeting should go on for more than 2 hours at the very most. If a discussion becomes lengthy or starts going round in circles, summarise where there is common agreement, then ask where you want to go from there.

11. *Summarise* the outcome/decision at the end of each agenda item and who agreed to do what. This confirms the message for everyone and makes it easier for the person taking notes.

12. *End the meeting on time.* Thank everyone for coming and their contributions and confirm the time and place of the next meeting.

13. *Produce action notes* with a named lead and the agreed timescale, either as part of the minutes but highlighted in bold or as a separate action plan with headings 'Decision', 'Action', 'Who By' and 'Date'.

14. *NEVER take notes and chair the meeting at the same time.* Always appoint a minutes or note taker at the beginning of each meeting if you have no administrative support.

LEARN TO LET GO THROUGH DELEGATION

Delegation is not about dumping the job onto someone else. Nobody likes working for someone who gives them all the rotten jobs. Delegation is about giving someone the responsibility and authority to carry out some work for you that is geared towards aiding their personal development.

Do not delegate jobs where failure to deliver would cause immense problems and don't delegate jobs that may be beyond the person's skills and abilities. The basic rules of good delegation are to:

- present the task as an opportunity or challenge
- ensure the individuals are fully aware of what is required of them – a written brief may be advisable
- identify areas where they will need support or further training
- ensure or give the individuals the appropriate authority to carry out what is required to complete the job
- agree timescales
- give feedback to enable them to learn from the process.

Remember that you still take full responsibility for the completion of the job. When you ask someone to do something for you, you are delegating, not abdicating your responsibility.

DELEGATION TO HEALTH CARE ASSISTANTS

The changing workforce today means that a greater number of nursing duties
are being delegated to health care assistants (HCAs). Some nurses have difficulty
with this concept and resort to delegating tasks such as doing the observations or
emptying catheter bags. This is not true delegation. These nurses are compensating
for their fear that nobody can do the job as well as they can. Proper delegation means
giving responsibility for the care of the patient, not individual tasks. The nurse should
continue to oversee patient care and remain accountable for it.

HCAs cannot learn and develop if their work is based on delegated tasks. In the long
term, delegation of patient-centred care instead of task-centred care will help develop
the skills and competences of HCAs. Nurses need to feel confident in their skills to be
able to trust them with the increased responsibilities. However, if they do not practise
true delegation, how will HCAs develop the required skills? (See also p. 85).

The art of true delegation is to enhance a person's development. Delegation is
probably one of the most important skills that both you and your staff should develop.

ARE YOU STILL DOING THE JOB YOU WERE PROMOTED FROM?

It is not uncommon for ward managers to find that they are still doing many aspects of
their old job in addition to their new responsibilities. Just because you are good at your
job of being a clinical nurse does not mean that you should continue to take a patient
caseload each shift. You are now in a position in which you oversee patient care rather
than actually carrying it out yourself. Your priority has now changed to ensuring your
team have the appropriate skills to be able to deliver that same high standard of care.

It is difficult to let go but if you want to develop in your role as ward manager,
you cannot do so unless you delegate your old role.

DELEGATING TO YOUR DEPUTY

A major aspect of your role is to ensure your deputy develops the appropriate
skills to be able to replace you at times of annual leave, sickness and when or if you
leave your job. As with your staff, don't delegate parts of a project in the form of
tasks – delegate the whole project. If you are going to delegate the investigation of
a complaint or serious incident, for example, don't ask them just to investigate and
report their findings to you. Give them the responsibility and authority to deal with
the whole thing, including writing the patient response or incident report. Your role
will be to provide support, advice and guidance throughout.

DELEGATE EFFECTIVELY

When delegating a task, make sure the person understands what is expected of
them. Get them to repeat it to you. Write down the objectives to ensure you agree

what needs to be done, the limits, and ensure the other person has full authority and training if required for carrying out the task.

Delegate gradually, without being too daunting. For example:

> 'Susan, would you like to have the chance to develop your skills in investigating formal complaints? We've had a letter from a patient about a couple of incidents that happened a few weeks ago. I'd like you to have a go at leading the investigation. I'll go through the process with you and will make sure you have some extra time out to devote to this. You'll have the opportunity to learn how to write a formal response too.'

Take a back seat while they are carrying out the work, making sure they know you are happy to support them if needed. Praise them if they are successful. If the task has not been completed to the correct standard, it is usually because the person has not fully understood what was required of them. Always give constructive feedback; that is, praise them for things done well and identify areas for improvement if they had to do a similar task in future.

BE PROACTIVE

UNDER-PROMISE AND OVER-DELIVER

A reputation for delivering on time earns you the reputation of being dependable. The only way you can do this is to ensure that you are not over-optimistic when setting deadlines. If you are asked to investigate and report on an incident within 48 hours, say you will need 5 days in order to gather the information, then set about getting the report done over the next 2–3 days. If you hand it in on day 3, people will be impressed, whereas if you had agreed to try and do it within 48 hours and then handed it in on day 3, your work would have been late. Setting a longer deadline date also reduces the pressure when you have any unforeseen setbacks.

Do the same when promising things to your team. If you say you should hopefully have the roster done by Tuesday, your staff will be expecting it done by then. They will not be happy if you produce the final roster on Thursday. However, if you say you will have it ready after the weekend and then produce it on Thursday, your staff will be under the impression that you are incredibly efficient.

DON'T PUT THINGS OFF

Avoid putting tasks off because you believe they will be difficult. They often turn out to be easier than you think. Even if they are not easy, start early and you have the time to spend sorting out the difficulties. You can also renegotiate the deadline if necessary.

Always begin reports early. Write an outline to start you off for reports, complaints responses and incident investigations (see Ch. 12). This will help guide you and stop you worrying about what needs to be done. If you don't do this immediately, you will end up putting it off by finding more important things to do, like welcoming interruptions to your office!

ASK FOR HELP

Ward managers tend to work in isolation and are often expected to get on with things. Remember that you have been trained clinically and all this managerial and paperwork stuff is new to you. It all needs to be learned through experience. And you cannot learn if you struggle to do everything by yourself. You'll pick up bad habits, which can then become normal practice.

If you have been delegated a piece of work to do and don't know where to start, go back to the person who delegated it and ask. If you get stuck halfway through the piece of work, go back and ask again. It doesn't matter if you feel a fool. Who cares? Next time you do a similar piece of work you will have learned through previous experience rather than having to struggle all over again.

KEEP YOUR PAPERWORK ORGANISED

Keeping your paperwork organised will make you feel as if you have more control over your work. Your aim is to complete as much work as possible in your 7.5-hour day, then when you go home you have earned the right to relax and do your own thing with your family and friends. The important thing is to have your time away from work for *you*. 'You work to live, not live to work.'

ACTION POINTS

- Define your workload and liaise with your manager to review it if you find that your commitments add up to more than 150 hours per month.
- Organise your office space and write everything you need to do on one 'to-do' list
- Reprioritise your 'to-do' list each day.
- Book all your annual leave at the start of each year. Try not to leave more than 3 months between each leave break.
- Allocate a set time each day to deal with your e-mails, ensuring that someone has proxy access to deal with them in your absence.
- When doing office work, ensure that you are not interrupted and keep your staff informed about the work you are doing.
- Don't get bogged down reading documents in detail. Scan or speed read them.
- Cut out all unnecessary meetings that do not benefit you, the team or your patients.
- When delegating work, ensure it is always a learning opportunity. Make sure your team do the same.
- From now on, always make sure you under-promise and over-deliver.

APPENDIX 2.1

EXAMPLE OF TERMS OF REFERENCE FOR A MEETING

DELAYED DISCHARGE MEETINGS

Terms of reference

Purpose:

To reduce the number of delayed discharges by making improvements to the overall patient discharge process.

Terms:

- Members of the meeting include the following list. Those who cannot attend are required to send an appropriate representative from their area.
- If a member misses more than three meetings in a row, the group will automatically assume that person has resigned.
- Agenda items to be with the secretary 5 days before the meeting date.
- Meetings will be held on the first and third Monday of each month, starting promptly at 2 pm and finishing at 3 pm.
- Latecomers will be expected to enter quietly and not attempt to interrupt the group by making apologies. The meeting will not be interrupted to update latecomers.
- Anyone who needs to leave early must make this known before the meeting starts.
- The first agenda item is to collate any other business (AOB), which is for emergency or short information items. The only points allowed under AOB will be those that were raised and agreed at the start.
- The second agenda item will always be to check the progress of action points from the previous meeting.

CREATE A POSITIVE WORKING ENVIRONMENT

What motivates a nurse to want to do well and to achieve more when they are at work? More money perhaps? Well, money's always welcome, but nurses have probably not chosen their vocation to earn lots of money. They have entered the profession for a different reason: to be able to make a difference to people's lives.

So why have so many become so demotivated? The answer probably has a lot to do with the fact that they feel less able to make that difference in people's lives.

Helping your team feel they are making a difference is an important element of the ward manager's role. And poor leadership can leave teams feeling low about their ability to achieve anything. Work becomes unsatisfying and frustrating. When individuals feel unempowered, they can lose confidence in themselves and lack self-esteem. Much of the research shows that increasing people's self-worth and confidence at work in achieving things is a great motivator. Teams under constant stress are rarely able to motivate themselves over a long period. They need a motivating environment and it is the role of the ward manager to create that environment.

PLAN AHEAD

Any group of health professionals working together can be viewed as a team. To be able to work together effectively and make the most of each others' skills, they need to be working towards the same goals. Your job is to create a motivating environment to enable your team to flourish. Take a good look at your team now:

1. Are there any problems with lateness and/or sickness?
2. Are any of your staff displaying inappropriate or unprofessional behaviour (e.g. flouting the uniform policy, sloppiness, defensiveness or showing an uncaring attitude)?
3. Are there problems between some members of the team who don't get on?
4. Are there individuals who persistently moan about things?
5. Are problems continually being discussed without any effective action ever taken?
6. Are they not particularly bothered about what is going on elsewhere in the organisation?
7. Have any cliques formed within the team?

If you answered yes to any of the above questions, it's a sign that you should probably be doing more to create a positive working environment. Behaviours like those are common in many working environments, but in poor working environments can take on a life of their own and interfere with the team's productivity.

Tackling individuals about these problems may not make much difference unless you have team objectives, communicate effectively and ensure you know the particular strengths of each individual within your team. These three elements are mentioned in most leadership and management textbooks, but tend to be submerged in various models, theories and jargon.

TEAM OBJECTIVES

What are your team's aspirations? What do your team want to change or improve on your ward? You probably know what *you* want and where you are heading, but have you any idea what your team want? Have you sat down with them all and asked them?

Some ward managers will say how they share their vision and goals with their team and keep them fully informed. This is a very 'top-down' autocratic approach. It would be far better to work *with* your team and establish some clear goals about what you want to aim for together. You may think that your main aim is to ensure patients get good quality care with proper discharge planning, but the main aim of your team may be to get home on time and stop having to stay late after each shift. This is not going to make for effective team working. For a team to co-operate with each other and work hard, it is better to agree your top priorities together.

COMMUNICATE EFFECTIVELY

Some think that being an effective communicator is to keep the team fully informed through regular meetings and perhaps using a communication book, which staff have to sign to prove they have read (and to cover themselves from staff saying 'no one told me'). This is effective *one-way* information giving, not effective communication. Effective communication should be *two-way* and that involves really hearing what others have to say and giving feedback.

Spend time listening to what your staff have to say. This sounds easy but it isn't. People tend to take the easy way out and give advice, opinions or relate a similar experience of their own and say what they did.

In addition to listening effectively, try and ensure that everyone receives regular feedback on how they are doing. Tell your staff when they have done something well and when they have not. It does not take as much time as listening but can reap rewards in terms of staff performance.

KNOW YOUR TEAM WELL

Once you know the individuals in your team, you can enable them to work on their strengths and to be aware of each other's weaknesses. Try not to focus on improving a person's weaknesses unless it involves clinical competences that need to be met. Focus on their strengths; that way they can only get better. Everyone has different strengths that they can contribute to their team.

Make it your personal plan from now on to focus on the three issues described above. It takes up too much time and energy to motivate each individual and will rarely work if you do not have a motivating environment. Focus instead on creating a positive working environment, which is the essence of being a good leader.

SET MEANINGFUL OBJECTIVES WITH YOUR TEAM

Some managers spend many hours with their staff facilitating discussions about their values and beliefs. From these, they produce a written mission statement or ward philosophy. It used to be the 'fashionable' thing to do. The ward philosophy would then be laminated and put up on the wall at the entrance to the ward. Some still do this. Does anyone ever read these things? I'm not so sure.

However, your team does need to work towards some sort of shared vision in order to be able to work well together and work hard. This 'shared vision' can be written down in the form of agreed priorities or objectives reflecting everyone's views on what constitutes a good working environment, and ultimately good patient care.

FIND OUT WHAT YOUR TEAM WANTS

It is a good idea to set shared objectives each year with the team. Ideally, it would be nice to get all the team together at once, but impossible when you have to cover a ward 24 hours a day, 7 days a week. So conduct two separate meetings with half the team attending the first one and half attending the second one. It is important that every single one of your staff is involved, so even three or four meetings may be necessary to allow for sickness, annual leave and emergencies.

At each meeting, ask your staff where they all want to be as a team in a year's time. Ask them which aspects of work they are dissatisfied with and what they would like to change. Values and beliefs may also be discussed and debated as your team aim to clarify what their mutual goals are. Remember to really listen to what they are saying and try not to impose your views. You may get a list looking something like the following:

- to get off work on time
- to have enough pillows for all the patients
- to reduce the paperwork required on admission
- to stop being hassled by the matron and bed manager about the bed state
- to know more about what is going on in the rest of the organisation
- to get more staff on the team
- to have food available when patients return from surgery or get cancelled
- to be able to get proper breaks off the ward at night.

Be careful to make sure the goals are congruent with the organisational goals. If, for example, your team would like to set up a post-discharge telephone helpline for patients and it is not part of your organisation's contract with the purchaser, then it cannot be part of your yearly objectives (although it could be an objective to add to the business plan next year).

You may prefer to start your meeting by getting the group to brainstorm ideas about what they want. Write each point up on a whiteboard or flipchart, then discuss and agree which are the top three or four priorities. Alternatively, you could ask everyone to identify his or her own top three personal priorities and get each one of the team to put a mark against each of these on the whiteboard or flipchart. Once everyone has done this, you should be able to see at a glance what the team's top priorities are, i.e. the objectives with most marks against them.

DEVELOP A TEAM ACTION PLAN

Once the main objectives have been agreed, your next step is to agree actions to achieve them. If, for example, the team's main objective is to get off work on time at the end of each shift, possible actions could include:

● reviewing the handover system to make it shorter, e.g. taped handover
● giving health care assistants (HCAs) more training to take on extra roles
● changing shift times to coincide with busier periods
● putting in a business case for an extra member of staff.

Make sure that the meeting is solution focused, not problem-focused. If you allow the team to focus on the problem, discussions tend to go around in circles and can easily devolve into whingeing sessions. By looking at possible solutions, you are focusing their minds on what they can do, not what they can't.

Ensure the actions are SMART, i.e. Specific, Measurable, Achievable, Realistic and have a Timetable. The final agreed action plan should then be reviewed regularly with the team together. Some of the objectives can even be incorporated into induction programmes and performance appraisals.

Having a set vision of where you and your team want to be in a year's time is crucial to effective team working. It is an essential but frequently overlooked part of good leadership.

BE A GOOD LISTENER

Few health care professionals have had specific training in listening skills. Sometimes rather than getting someone to talk, they can end up achieving quite the opposite. Your staff need to be sure that you really understand and are interested in what they are saying.

FOCUS ON UNDERSTANDING WHAT PEOPLE ARE SAYING

Sometimes when listening to others we do not really hear what they are saying. While the person is speaking, we tend to:

● think about a similar experience that we have had ourselves
● try to see things from our own point of view
● think of answers or suggestions.

We then spend time relating our own similar experience, telling them our opinion or giving advice based on what we think is going on. In essence, we have not really listened to them at all. Take a look at the following example of a conversation between a staff nurse (SN) and ward manager (WM):

> SN: 'Sister, can I have a word with you? I'm having a problem with the porters. They are reluctant to take our patients to X-ray. The X-ray porter is on long-term sick leave and they say they are not X-ray porters.'

WM: 'I've had this problem before. I called the head porter and he sorted it. Try him and see what happens.'

One week later:

SN: 'I called the head porter last week like you said, and he said he would speak to them, but nothing seems to have changed. They still won't listen to me.'

WM: 'I think they are just being obstructive. Leave it to me, I'll go and speak to them.'

You probably recognise these types of responses. The ward manager is well intended, but is basically interpreting what the staff nurse is saying and giving advice based on her own previous experience ('I've had this problem before') and opinions ('I think they are just being obstructive'). She has not really listened so cannot really understand what the issue is. Now consider the following scenario:

SN: 'Sister, can I have a word with you? I'm having a problem with the porters. They are reluctant to take our patients to X-ray. The X-ray porter is on long-term sick leave and they say they are not X-ray porters.'

WM: 'You sound really frustrated.'

SN: 'Yes I am. I've tried talking to them but they just ignore me. I'm not sure if I'm going about it the right way.'

WM: 'How do you mean?'

SN: 'Well, I do have a tendency to apologise every time I call them. I feel as though I'm asking them to do me a personal favour, but it is their job.'

WM: 'You mean perhaps you are asking them too nicely?'

SN: 'Yes, I suppose I am really. Perhaps I should be just a bit more direct when I call them, rather than beginning with an apology.'

WM: 'That might be an idea. Is there anything you would like me to do?'

SN: 'No, not yet. I'll try and be a bit more direct from now on when I call them. If it doesn't work, I'll let you know.'

By spending just a little more time really listening to what the staff nurse is saying, the ward manager has been able to find out what the real issue is. Giving advice won't help matters unless you find out what the problem really is. It only clears up what appears on the surface. In the first scenario, the staff nurse would have been left frustrated and probably with reduced confidence. Before being given a chance to go through the issue, the ward manager is taking the issue off her hands and dealing with it herself. If the staff nurse had a problem with assertiveness, the first approach would only serve to exacerbate that problem.

Try and spend just a little more time listening to your staff. It will not only help you to really understand the problem, but also, when given the opportunity to explain things, staff often come up with the answers themselves during the process. It helps if you can continually reflect back their questions:

SN: 'What can I do?'

WM: 'What do you think you could do?' or 'What are your options?'

If you are one of those managers who often has a queue of staff waiting to see you, try the above technique. It gradually enables your staff to take the initiative and think for themselves instead of having to rely on you.

FEEDBACK WITH SINCERITY

THANKING STAFF AT THE END OF THE SHIFT IS NOT ENOUGH

Some managers will say they always thank their staff at the end of each shift, but giving out a general thank you is not the best way of giving feedback. Your staff will not know specifically what they have done well. Giving general thanks will not improve people's performance. It could simply be seen as acknowledging their presence. One could well be saying 'Thank you for turning up today!' General feedback can also be rather patronising. The manager is saying that everyone has done well but what about the one or two who have not? There are often some people who have worked harder than others. They will not feel genuinely appreciated. They may feel that their hard work has gone unnoticed if those who did not work so hard are included in the general feedback.

Be genuine

People need genuine feedback to know what they are doing well and which areas need to be improved, and they should not have to wait until their appraisal to find this out. Make it an aim to provide some sort of feedback to each member of your team on a daily basis. For example, if a member of your staff spotted a patient deteriorating and took corrective action, then tell them, 'Well done. I'm impressed with the way you handled that. You did well to lay the patient flat immediately and increase the fluids before calling me'.

If you give feedback like this, your staff will know what they did well and ensure they do it next time. Just saying 'well done' generates very little in terms of improving performance.

USE GENERAL FEEDBACK AS AN OPPORTUNITY FOR OTHERS TO LEARN

Try to ensure you give positive feedback in front of others. It not only makes the person feel good, it helps the rest of the team to improve their performance too. They are learning what they should be doing themselves in such circumstances. You also need to ensure members of your staff know when they have not done so well. But never criticise! You want to keep your staff motivated. Always remember the golden rule: with any feedback, whether negative or positive, the person receiving it must end up feeling good about themselves.

How to give negative feedback

Treat negative feedback as an area for improvement but make sure it is sandwiched within lots of positive feedback. For example, 'Well done. You did well to lay the patient flat immediately and increase the fluids before calling me. Do remember next time to ensure you chart the observations, but overall I am impressed with the way you handled the situation'.

The person receiving such feedback will make a mental note to chart the observations down in future but the most important thing is that their self-esteem remains intact.

It's your role as a leader to increase the confidence and self-esteem of each and every member of your team. They will end up a lot more motivated. You know yourself how good you feel when you receive constructive feedback. When giving any type of negative feedback, make sure that:

1. *You are objective, never subjective.* In other words, stick to the facts and leave out any personal opinions. Saying, for example, 'You don't seem to be prioritising your work as well as you could be' will be far more effective and less damaging than saying: 'Your work is sloppy and unprofessional'.
2. *You listen carefully and try to enable the person to come to their own conclusion about what they can do to improve.* You can give them information and share ideas, but if you get them to think of the answer, they will be more likely to put this into action.

PEOPLE RECEIVE FEEDBACK EVEN IF YOU DO NOT GIVE IT

If you do not give regular feedback, your staff will be left to guess what you are thinking. They will note your body language, listen to gossip or look to others less experienced for feedback, which may not be appropriate. Be proactive and make sure all feedback is given in a positive manner.

KNOW YOUR STAFF WELL

Aim to have an individual knowledge of each and every member of your team that you work with and directly supervise. Recognise the strengths each person brings to the team. For example, if there is someone in your team who is really popular and networks well, ensure that person represents your team on important groups within your organisation. They can tell everyone about the good practice on your ward and at the same time bring relevant information back to your team. It does not just have to be you or your deputy who attends meetings. Use the talents of others to the team's advantage.

FOCUS ON STRENGTHS, NOT WEAKNESSES

If you enable the individuals in your team to develop their strengths, you will consistently improve the whole team. Focusing on a person's weaknesses can serve to demoralise and reduce self-esteem. Some say that weaknesses should be seen as 'areas for improvement'. However, if you put too much focus on improving weaknesses, a person's strengths may not be used to their full potential. Their strengths can become weaker, and their weaknesses can be improved. The result could be that the person becomes average and you end up with a team of nurses turning out average work. Work on the individual strengths within the team and you could have a better than average team.

DEVOTE EQUAL TIME TO EVERY MEMBER OF YOUR TEAM

Try and treat each of your staff fairly. When you first become a manager, you may notice that your staff fall into one of two groups. The first group are those that are naturally enthusiastic and motivated. They are generally ambitious, love their job and want to get on. Staff that fall into the second group are those that fulfil the basic requirements of their job but are unwilling to take on any additional responsibilities or get involved in any new initiatives.

It is easy to fall into the trap of devoting more time and effort to staff in the first group. These people want to get on so you naturally feel they deserve more of your attention. If you do this, you run the risk of creating resentment and ultimately you are discriminating against the other members of your team. It is advisable to ensure that all receive an equal share of your time and resources.

In the same way, try to ensure that you do not personally put extra time and effort into helping a member of your staff who needs additional education and supervision. Allocate one of your senior staff to assist. Doing it yourself will only take your attention away from the rest of the team. You may be the most skilled and experienced member of the team but it does not mean that you are the only one who can deal with problems. Your role is to empower others to do so. That way, you will ensure that they become more skilled and experienced.

BE INVOLVED IN ALL APPRAISALS

Make sure you are involved in and sign off all performance appraisals for your team. This does not mean you have to do them all. That would not be a good use of your time. You just need to make sure that you are continuously aware of where your staff are heading in terms of career development and where their strengths and weaknesses lie.

The development needs of your staff are paramount. Sending them away on courses is a very small part of their development. Being aware of their needs and strengths will ensure that you are able to build on them on a regular basis during the working shift.

NEVER TALK DISAPPROVINGLY OF OTHERS

It doesn't matter how much someone frustrates, annoys or upsets you, try not to let your team see this. They will not respect you for talking about others in such a manner. Losing the respect of your team will make your job a lot harder than it already is.

YOUR MANAGER(S)

Be careful about using the term 'the management'. You are part of 'the management'. You shouldn't create the impression that it is 'us and them'. If you say things like 'I can't let you do that because the management won't let me', you may create the impression that you are weak and have no influence.

If you feel your own line manager is not particularly good at their job, keep that frustration to yourself. Your team needs to feel confident in you and the rest of the organisation. They need to feel that you are influential and that, together, you and the organisation have their best interests at heart. Work it through with your mentor if you just feel the need to moan and whinge about any managers. Talk to your spouse, partner or friends with no professional connections. Just keep it out of the work environment. The informal 'grapevine' in large public organisations means that very little remains confidential for long.

TALKING ABOUT PROBLEMATIC STAFF

You will always have colleagues, managers and even friends who do not do their jobs properly, behave in ways you don't like or are unable to manage their priorities, thereby creating more work or problems for you. That's life. But while moaning about others may make you feel better for a few minutes, it's doubtful it's going to achieve anything except damage how others see you. If you find yourself moaning about others, make yourself stop and think, 'What can I do about it?' Then take action. If you can't think of an answer, then don't moan. It's a waste of your precious time. People see those that moan and whinge excessively as idle and petty. It can give the impression that they do not have enough work to do. That is not the impression you want to give.

Also, be careful not to talk about a member of your staff with another, either in confidence or in front of others. If any members of your team hear you making disparaging remarks about one of their colleagues, all they will think is 'What is being said about me when my back is turned?' You risk losing their trust in you.

LOOK FOR THE POSITIVE IN OTHERS

Make it your mission to always see the positive in people. Don't dwell on the negatives. If you hear members of your team talking negatively about their colleagues, either:

1. *Turn the conversation around by mentioning the individual's positive aspects.*
   It usually has the effect of making the negative talker feel guilty and they tend to stop, or
2. *Ask them, 'Have you told x how you feel?'* More often than not, they will not have done so, and again it will usually stop the moaning. They will understand that what you are really saying is, 'If you can't tell this person to their face, then it's not very nice to talk about it behind their back, is it?' but in a nice kind of way!

As their leader, you are your team's role model. If you are consistent in your manner and are never seen to moan or talk disapprovingly of others, your team will hopefully take note and follow in your footsteps.

GET YOUR STAFF TO TAKE MORE RESPONSIBILITY

Empowering staff is not as easy as it sounds. You have to be very confident in the skills of your team. It means that you can no longer have full knowledge of what is going on. When you have overall 24-hour responsibility for the welfare of the patients on your ward, it is difficult to devolve responsibility to others. But in order to allow individuals to flourish in your team, you have to let them learn from their experiences, including their mistakes. There are still some wards where the nurse-in-charge has a list of things to do for the patients, such as:

- following up the consultant ward round
- sorting out some delayed discharges
- ensuring wound swabs/urine samples are taken
- ensuring pre-operative patients are all prepared for theatre.

This is a very top-down approach. The nurses who have been allocated their patients, either through patient allocation, team nursing or primary nursing, should be wholly responsible for everything to do with their patient on that shift. If a patient's discharge needs sorting, it should be by them and nobody else. The role of the nurse-in-charge is to assist them should they need it. If there are things to be sorted from ward rounds, for example, it is the patient's nurse who should be dealing with these things, not the nurse-in-charge.

'Nurses only have time to do the basic care'

Some managers say their nurses don't have the time to sort out things like the patient's discharge because they need the time to care for the patient; however, sorting out things like discharge arrangements or implementing changes from the ward round *are* all part of caring for the patient. Spending the shift undertaking delegated nursing tasks rather than having responsibility for total patient care is very unsatisfying. Doing it day in and day out is boring and may only serve to produce apathy in your staff. In this case, care is not patient-centred, it is centred with the nurse-in-charge.

ALLOW YOUR STAFF TO DO MORE FOR THEIR ALLOCATED PATIENTS

Having full responsibility for all aspects of the patient's care is the main way that your staff will learn and develop. It is also highly satisfying and motivating to be totally in charge of all care for a group of patients.

The role of the nurse-in-charge should be to support and coordinate the team, not take over or delegate parts of the care. Nurses and support workers who are given full responsibility for a group of patients are far more likely to be satisfied in their work than those who are expected to carry out only the basic nursing tasks for their patients. The latter is not team nursing or patient allocation, it is task allocation, and can be very demotivating. But you have to trust your staff and that is not easy. You have to trust that they will sort out the patient's discharge arrangements, take that urgent wound swab, speak to the relatives, etc. You also have to support them when they make mistakes. The key is to ensure you support them to learn from their mistakes and for you or the nurse-in-charge to be available and help out when needed. Your team are more likely to develop and flourish in such an environment.

HAVE A SYSTEM FOR DEALING WITH PATIENTS' VISITORS

Being the relative of a patient can be an incredibly anxious and stressful experience. To leave your loved one in a vulnerable state in the hands of strangers in a strange environment is not easy. But to enter that environment and see one or two nurses rushing around looking hassled and overworked does not inspire one's confidence. Worse still, having to wait for ages to grab someone's attention only to get answers like 'Sorry, she's not my patient' or 'I've just come back after days off' or 'He hasn't had his bath/wound dressed/drip changed because we are too short staffed' is not very encouraging. And people wonder why relatives get so angry and demanding!

MAKE YOUR WARD WELCOMING

Hospitals are unfamiliar environments to most people. Entering a ward can be an unnerving experience. Few wards indicate where visitors should go or to whom they should speak. Nerves are easily frayed and tempers easily lost. You do not want to expose your staff to any unnecessary abuse or harassment.

Don't blame the relatives; first look at your environment. Imagine being a stranger entering the ward. Is it indicated clearly where you should go and to whom you should speak?

You may have an information/photo board at the entrance to the ward, showing who your staff are, what their uniforms mean and perhaps even how they are split into smaller teams. But is it clear which nurses are looking after which patients? If you have divided your staff into two teams such as red and blue, which are the red and blue beds? How can the relatives match the two? Do you have boards by the beds indicating which nurses are looking after the patients that day? If you don't, relatives will continually ask, causing unnecessary interruptions for your staff. If you make as much information as possible available at a glance, it will serve much to appease your visitors.

FIRST IMPRESSIONS ALWAYS COUNT

You want the visitors to be happy that your ward is well run and their relative is in safe hands. Despite the advent of primary nursing, team nursing and increased responsibility of staff nurses, relatives still see the ward manager, sister or charge nurse as the one who should know everything. It's advisable to ensure that the nurse-in-charge is available at visiting times. It can save so much angst. If you ensure they are around to talk to visitors and answer any queries, it will reassure people that they are in control of their work and do not look as if they cannot manage the demands. You need to give the impression and reassurance that the patients on your ward are in safe hands.

Obviously times have changed and you cannot know everything about every patient on your ward. The turnover of patients is too fast nowadays. However, you should know the basic details such as the patient's name and why they are in hospital. Refer them to the appropriate nurse looking after the patient if further information is required. If the member of staff looking after the patient is an inexperienced nurse or an HCA, then stay and support them in giving the information.

BE CAREFUL WITH PATIENT CONFIDENTIALITY

Care plans and evaluations left at the end of patients' beds are inviting for the perusal of visitors. If possible, try and leave them with the patient at the head of the bed or in their locker. Keep all records behind the reception desk if the patient is not in a position to keep them confidential, such as confused patients or those just returned from surgery.

Use your common sense with regards to the Data Protection Act. There is little wrong with patient name boards at the head or end of the bed. The risk of not having one can be far greater in terms of mixing up patients' treatments. Just don't add the little extras like 'diabetic' for everyone to see.

DEAL WITH CONFLICT

No matter how happy or motivating you make the working environment, you will always come up against difficult people and difficult situations. Don't ignore these situations or you will allow them to blow up out of all proportion.

Whatever preventative steps you take, arguments may still occur between visiting relatives, health professionals and within your own team. The main rule is to take the argument away from the patients. If you catch staff having arguments or heated discussions in front of patients, take them elsewhere immediately and explain that the behaviour will not be tolerated on your ward. Support your senior staff in doing the same thing. They also need to gain the skills in dealing with conflict and not shy away from it.

DISCIPLINARY ACTION

Make sure you know your organisation's disciplinary policy. This outlines what constitutes unacceptable behaviour and the steps to take when such behaviour is displayed (see Ch. 4). Don't threaten disciplinary action. Disciplinary action can only be taken after a formal investigation.

If someone's behaviour is unacceptable under the terms of the disciplinary policy, seek advice from your human resources (HR) department about instigating a formal investigation. It is advisable to ensure you are familiar with what sorts of behaviour are not acceptable according to your organisation's policy. As the manager, you will have to make instant decisions in such situations. It is best to make sure that you have the appropriate knowledge to do so.

DON'T ALLOW DISAGREEMENTS TO GET OUT OF HAND

There are still some wards and departments in which some health professionals within a team do not speak to each other or don't get on. Allowing these situations to continue can have major knock-on effects:

1. It can reflect badly on the ward manager who has allowed it to get out of hand.
2. It may have a detrimental effect on the rest of the team who end up having to take sides.
3. It can affect the standards of patient care because people are not working together.

Don't allow it to happen on your ward. If you have a situation like this and feel unable to handle it, get help. Don't ignore it. You must do something about it. Not only that, you must be seen to do something about it. No team will respect a leader who cannot handle conflict. If you do not feel you have the skills, find someone who does and get them to support you through the process.

BULLYING OR HARASSMENT

If any of your staff are bullying or harassing others, you must also take action. It should not be tolerated under any circumstances. If you have a situation where someone like the bed manager or another health professional is behaving aggressively towards your staff, it is your duty to protect them. Consult your bullying and harassment policy and involve HR right from the beginning.

It is usually advisable in the first instance to help and support the individual to deal with the situation themselves. If you take over immediately, it may only serve to reduce their self-esteem even further. To be able to confront someone who is bullying or harassing them with your full support may give the individual a greater sense of satisfaction and self-worth. If it does not work, at least they will know they have tried.

NOT ALL CONFLICT IS DETRIMENTAL

Conflict at work is not always such a bad thing. In fact, if everyone insisted on smoothing things over and continually compromising their work in order to avoid causing fuss or arguments, things might never change. Maintaining the status quo is not always the best option. Encouraging people to speak up and confront people or situations that may be harmful for the patients should be encouraged. However, it's imperative to ensure your staff have the skills to do so (see Chs 12 and 13).

IMPLEMENT CLINICAL SUPERVISION

WHY HAVE CLINICAL SUPERVISION?

Nursing care and clinical treatments are continually changing and being updated. Unfortunately, getting a degree does not give nurses skills for life. A lot of nursing skills can only be gained through experience. Skills such as dealing with bereaved relatives, counselling a patient prior to disfiguring surgery or teaching a newly diagnosed diabetic how to give their own injections can only be perfected through practice. But they can only be perfected if the nurse has someone more experienced to help them reflect on their current practice.

ALL YOUR STAFF SHOULD HAVE ACCESS TO SOMEONE MORE EXPERIENCED

In an ideal world, a practice facilitator would be available at all times on the ward to work with individual staff to give advice, guidance and support, and ensure that they reflect and learn from their daily work. However, this is not an ideal world, so the next best thing is to ensure each member of your team has access to a more experienced member of staff whom they can learn from. It doesn't matter what you call it – mentorship, coaching, facilitation or clinical supervision. In essence, all members of your team should have access to a more experienced member of staff regularly to help them reflect and learn from their everyday experiences.

The most obvious and inexpensive way to do this is to ensure that each junior staff nurse is matched up with a more experienced senior staff nurse, *who is not a direct assessor or allocated to do their performance appraisal*. If the junior member thinks that what they are going to say may influence their performance appraisal, they may be reluctant to be open about their practice.

If you operate team nursing, it might be worth considering allocating each junior nurse a more senior nurse from the opposite team. That way at least there will be more chance of the two of them working the same shifts.

One-to-one or group supervision?

One-to-one clinical supervision is ideal but expensive. If you are allowing an hour per month for each individual member of your staff to have clinical supervision, it can prove to be very costly unless they can find time during the shift to go off somewhere quiet for an hour. A less expensive way of ensuring your team are learning from their experiences is through facilitated group supervision; in other words, having someone to facilitate a small group of staff to reflect and learn from their experiences together. Even if they discuss just one issue from one member of the group, the whole group are reflecting and learning from their colleague's experience.

CLINICAL SUPERVISION COURSES

Whether you decide on one-to-one or group supervision, you will need to ensure that the senior members of your team have the appropriate facilitation skills to help others to reflect and learn from their practice. Most organisations offer short courses on developing reflective skills or clinical supervision. It's well worth the investment.

As health care professionals, your staff have a duty to continually update themselves by reflecting and learning from their experience. As their manager, you have a duty to provide the right conditions for doing so.

ACTION POINTS

- Use your next few team meetings or arrange a couple of away days to identify your priorities as a team and agree specific team goals to achieve over the coming year.
- From now on, each time a member of staff comes to you with a concern, take time to really listen before giving advice.
- Give some specific feedback to each member of staff that works with you on your shift. Do this every shift.
- Each time you find yourself moaning or whingeing about something or someone, stop yourself and concentrate on finding a solution to the problem.
- Consider how your team are allocating patients. Are all staff being given the opportunity to have full responsibility for their patients?
- Put up an information board for visitors at the entrance to the ward or review the one you have to ensure it is clear where to go and who to see.
- Read your local disciplinary policy to ensure you are familiar with what your organisation defines as unacceptable behaviour.
- Find out what courses are available for the senior members of your staff to develop their clinical supervision skills.

MANAGE STAFF PERFORMANCE

Managing staff is an important part of the ward manager's role. As described in the previous chapter, it entails keeping them informed, involved and empowered to make decisions for themselves. If you are having problems with the performance of individuals in your team, read through Chapter 3 first and ask yourself if you have done enough to create a positive working environment. However, having done that, you may still have to deal with inappropriate or unacceptable behaviour from individuals from time to time, that is, any behaviour that disrupts your team or is detrimental to the welfare of the patients. It may also include behaviour that is unlawful or unethical.

Any behaviour that disrupts or upsets others should be 'nipped in the bud'. Allowing it to continue could affect staff morale. You owe it to the rest of the team to deal with any individual behavioural issues swiftly and proactively. It's essential to know your policies and know how to use them and have the skills to deal with such circumstances without having to resort to the formal route if at all possible.

GET TO KNOW YOUR HR ADVISOR

As they are very labour intensive, good staff management is of great importance to health care organisations. This means they typically have large human resources (HR) departments to help managers do a better job.

Your allocated HR advisor is there to help and guide you, so it makes sense to use this expert advice. Their role is to *advise* you on the appropriate policies and procedures which set out the expectations of your organisation, and the formal steps you can take if staff behaviour becomes unacceptable.

ARRANGE REGULAR MEETINGS

It is wise to build up a good professional relationship with your HR advisor right from the start, rather than wait until you need their advice. Meet them regularly, once a month or so, to go through any issues and potential problems, and to keep them up-to-date with how your team are getting on. They will become familiar with how you manage your ward and the sorts of problems you are dealing with each day. If you have to deal with a major disciplinary matter, it is much easier to take advice from someone you know and trust rather than someone you have hardly met.

In addition, if your HR advisor is called to help deal with a staff issue while you are on 'days off' or annual leave, they are more likely to be aware of the background to the problem and be able to give appropriate advice, based on your style of management. By keeping your HR advisor informed, you can also rest assured that your senior staff will be well supported in your absence.

LEARNING FROM EXPERIENCE

Like you, most HR advisors are also learning from each new experience, but if they do not have experience of a particular problem, they do have direct access to the HR director for advice and guidance. They also gain experience of issues from other departments, such as disciplinary hearings, which they can share with you.

Having insight into general HR issues will help you deal with future problems as and when they occur. And you can develop the appropriate wisdom to know when to take risks on behalf of your staff.

CONSULT THE POLICY AT THE INFORMAL STAGE

Don't wait to familiarise yourself with the appropriate policy until the point where you feel the issue needs to be dealt with formally. This is often too late. It's advisable to see what is advised at the informal stage. This can help prevent the need to go on to the formal stage.

Most policies set out what to do at the informal stage. If you do not deal with the problem informally as set out in the appropriate policy, you may not be able to proceed to the next stage if the situation does not improve. Your HR advisor is there to support and guide you through all stages when dealing with a staff problem, but only if you require them to. It is not their job to 'tell' you what to do. You are the manager and it's you alone who takes the consequences for decisions regarding management performance.

GET TO KNOW EACH OTHER'S TEAMS

Invite your HR advisor to help you with interviewing staff. Involve them in your team meetings where you set goals together and devise action plans to deal with ward issues. They will note how you are leading your team and perhaps even share your good practice with their colleagues. It will help increase the profile of your ward within the organisation.

When you do meet your HR advisor, try and make sure you go to see them in their department rather than have them coming to see you all the time. You will become familiar with how the HR department works, the different staff and their roles, including the reception staff. It helps to know who does what and to be able to greet them on first name terms. This improves access for when you may require their advice in future. It also helps you to know the different skills and attributes everyone has in the team. You can then contact them directly rather than just blindly phoning the HR department.

WRITE EVERYTHING DOWN
KEEP FILE NOTES

Try and get into the habit of keeping brief notes of face-to-face meetings or phone conversations where performance may be an issue. This saves so much time in the future when trying to recall what was said, where and when. Keeping notes before incidents happen will also help enormously. It is too late afterwards to remember that you had several conversations with a person who denies that you mentioned something. If you keep file notes, they will aid you in remembering what was said and when, rather than hazy details.

The file notes can be kept either in the person's personal file or a file of your own. They can help months or even years later when an incident involving a member of your staff occurs and you are asked if it was a problem earlier.

Don't focus on negative events

Don't just note negative things that may be useful if an incident occurs subsequently. It is also helpful to make file notes when the member of staff does something positive and is praised for doing so. All the file notes you keep about staff will be a useful aid when you come to doing their appraisal as well as any future references.

File notes save time

It can be difficult to fit the writing of file notes into a busy schedule but once you get into the habit you will find that they save you time. Keep notes throughout your day. Make a file note of any meetings you have had either with staff as a group or in one-to-one meetings. Keep the file notes short and to the point. Briefly note any actions agreed. These notes can prove useful as the basis for the next meeting or review of progress.

What you can and can't include in file notes

Never write down anything derogatory or subjective, and never write down anything that you can't justify or substantiate at a later date. All staff have the right to see any documents within their organisation that have their name mentioned (Section 7 of the Data Protection Act, IC 1998). If you keep any notes about anyone, they should never contain anything that you would not want the person to see.

Be open and honest with your staff. Show them the file notes you make, or at least let them know that you will make a note of the conversation you have just had. The file notes enable you to:

- carry out better performance appraisals
- provide an accurate recording of events months or even years later if required
- write informed references for your staff
- provide information that would help in future decision making
- remind you of previous events
- help you to review progress of certain behaviours or events.

KEEP MEETING NOTES

When you attend any meetings, keep brief notes and share them with your team. Leave them on the coffee table in the staff room. Keep notes of all your own team meetings. You do not have to keep formal minutes of local team meetings. Write up some brief notes, which serve simply to keep your staff informed.

KEEP A STAFF COMMUNICATION BOOK AND NOTICE BOARD

It's a good idea to print off any important e-mails, new policies or procedures or any written communication that you receive which may affect your staff. Highlight any pertinent bits, particularly on minutes of meetings. It helps them to see quickly which parts of the documents they need to know, rather than being put off by the surrounding jargon.

Asking your staff to sign when a document has been read can be seen as a rather officious 'top-down' approach and could cause resentment. If you make sure the information is relevant to their day-to-day practice and highlight the relevant parts in any long documents, there is a greater chance that your staff will be motivated to read it rather than being 'told' to sign something.

MAKE APPRAISALS WORK

Don't take on too many appraisals. Some ward managers decide to carry out appraisals on every single member of their staff. This is very cumbersome and is certainly not an effective use of time. It allows little space for other senior staff to develop their skills in this area, and is a very top-down approach. It is advisable for the ward manager to select a few such as:

- the deputy ward manager(s), sisters and charge nurses
- one or two more experienced senior staff nurses
- the ward receptionist,

The deputy ward managers, sisters and charge nurses can do the staff nurse appraisals and the staff nurses can do the appraisals for the health care assistants. The ward manager, however, should see and countersign them all. That way, you can ensure that no-one is going off at a tangent and attending courses that have nothing to do with the needs of your wards, for example. It will also help you to support staff in the process of doing appraisals.

HOW TO APPROACH APPRAISALS

The purpose of formal appraisals is to enhance a person's development and skills to ensure they are meeting the goals of the team and the organisation. It is not meant to be a list of the individual's personal wants and needs. You should not be agreeing personal development plans or granting courses of study that are not congruent with the goals of your team or the organisation.

An individual's personal development plan should be based on three important documents:

1. The objectives of the organisation.
2. The objectives of your ward team.
3. The Knowledge and Skills Framework (KSF) (if working within the NHS).

WHY SOME PEOPLE DON'T LIKE APPRAISALS

Some people groan when you mention performance appraisals. This could be because they have had bad experiences of them in the past. The one thing that some managers do badly when appraising staff is simply that they take too long, or take them too seriously. After all, they should just be a simple summary which formally acknowledges everything you have said over the past year and sets objectives for the next year. That's all. If you are giving feedback to all members of staff regularly (see p. 49), then you should need no more than an hour at the very most to carry out a performance appraisal. If more than an hour is needed, then perhaps you need to ask yourself why. It can indicate that you are not spending enough time listening to your staff or, more importantly, giving regular feedback in between appraisals.

FORMALISING WHAT IS ALREADY KNOWN

An appraisal is not the time for discussing anything new. It should just be a formal confirmation of what both parties already know and have discussed on previous occasions. When you give constant feedback during the year, the appraisal should be easy to do and comfortable for both you and the appraisee.

Try not to postpone or cancel an appraisal unless absolutely necessary. It can be quite damaging in that it can give the impression to your staff that their appraisal is not important. To them, it is very important.

FIVE STEPS FOR A SUCCESSFUL APPRAISAL

Step 1: Self-assessment by appraisee

A few weeks before the appraisal, ask the appraisee to write down anything they would like to discuss and the objectives they would like to agree at appraisal. Most organisations provide a self-assessment form with questions to help stimulate their thoughts. They may also need to provide some evidence for their KSF requirements. Make sure you let the appraisee know that their notes/provisional evidence will be discussed with your line manager.

Step 2: Meet with your own line manager

Review the self-assessment form with your line manager to ensure the objectives are congruent with the organisation's objectives. They will be able to give advice about where else the appraisee can go for guidance and support in meeting the objectives, and any funding for development can be provisionally agreed.

Step 3: Carry out the appraisal

Your organisation will provide a specific appraisal form, usually based on the KSF. If possible, try to ensure you complete the form with the appraisee as part of the review rather than writing it up at a later date. It will save you a lot of time. Another good idea is to encourage the appraisee to write up the agreed objectives and action plan afterwards.

Remember to ensure that the appraisee should be encouraged to talk for as much of the time as possible (using the listening and feedback skills outlined in Ch. 3).

It's advisable to start off with a general discussion about how the past year has gone with regards to performance and development, followed by a review of the past year's objectives, followed by an agreement on next year's objectives and a personal development plan to meet those objectives. Remember that you don't have to focus on formal study or courses for development. Taking on projects with support and feedback can often be just as helpful.

Tips on reducing the paperwork for KSF:

- Focus on development needs and priorities, not every dimension.
- Avoid focusing on written evidence for each dimension. This does not have to be provided as you should both be able to refer to relevant actions and examples (The NHS Staff Council 2010).

Step 4: Agree the final appraisal document

Agree the final document with both the appraisee and your line manager. All three of you should sign it. The same goes for your own staff carrying out appraisals. It is advisable that you agree and sign all those that have been carried out within your team.

Step 5: Set a date for review

Mark in next year's diary when the next appraisal review is due. You may also want to set a date half way through the year to review the person's progress towards the agreed objectives.

ADAPT THE FORM TO THE APPRAISAL, NOT THE APPRAISAL TO THE FORM

Try not to focus too much on the actual form. It should be used as a guide. You don't have to fill in all the boxes, apart from the KSF final grades. Everyone is different and each appraisal will be different. If you focus on just filling in the form, the process can become overly bureaucratic. Your role is to help your staff remove the barriers to achieve success. Focusing on form filling is not being a good role model.

KNOW HOW TO HANDLE UNACCEPTABLE BEHAVIOUR

If a person's behaviour starts affecting others in the team and reducing morale, it becomes unacceptable and you need to take action.

First, make sure you address the problem behaviour early and when you are not angry about it. Never allow your feelings to colour your input or behaviour. If you are very angry or irritated, it is usually better to talk at a later time when you have calmed down. This makes sure that you can think and speak objectively and rationally.

Second, arrange to meet with the person as soon as possible. Leaving it will only add to their worry (and yours) and may cause them to become defensive and upset. Generally, it is advised that you try and deal with these things informally first. A good leader should 'protect' their staff from bureaucratic policies whenever possible.

GUIDELINES FOR CARRYING OUT THE FIRST MEETING

1. Don't set an open-ended meeting. It could go on for hours, especially if the staff member denies their behaviour is unacceptable. It's advisable to set a time limit on the discussion, and stick to it.
2. Ask them to go through with you their version of the events or incidents in question. Take the time to listen. Try to see their point of view and do not be defensive.
3. Once you have listened to their version, you can then give your assessment. Refer to facts only, not opinions. Respect their right to disagree with your assessment of the situation.
4. Keep the discussion focused on their behaviours. Don't let them blame personality or another person's actions. An example would be to say, '… that may be true about Jane, but we are here to discuss your behaviour'.
5. Summarise the discussion and the agreed actions clearly and succinctly at the end of the meeting.
6. Ensure the meeting is documented. Write up your notes in a factual, concise manner and agree an action plan with a clear timetable.
7. Both you and the employee must sign all documentation. Even if this is just a quick 10-minute discussion where the person agrees verbally to improve their behaviour, it should be documented.
8. Always try to end these meetings on a positive note. Remember the rules about giving feedback: positive, negative, and then positive (see p. 49).
9. It is very important to make sure you follow up the meeting. Arrange a date for review of progress. Hopefully the problem will be resolved and you will be able to give positive feedback.

DON'T ALLOW THE BEHAVIOUR TO CONTINUE

Do not allow the member of staff to continue to practise the unacceptable behaviour in question. If it does continue, despite your efforts, you may have to refer to the appropriate policy guidance. If you do not, the behaviour will only continue or worsen and the rest of your team will lose respect for your management abilities. They may even adopt such inappropriate behaviour themselves having seen that one person has got away with it. 'Nip it in the bud' and you will maintain a well-balanced team who respect your ability to manage situations rather than allowing them to get out of hand.

HANDLE POOR PERFORMANCE/INCOMPETENCE
WHAT EXACTLY IS INCOMPETENCE?

Before you label a member of your staff as incompetent, first ask yourself, 'How do I know that they are incompetent?' In other words, what criteria are you measuring them up against? Personal opinion is not sufficient. While you may think they are incompetent, another person may not.

Competence should be assessed with reference to the knowledge, skills and aptitudes required for the job you employed someone to do. In other words, you need to have very clear competences or standards against which you can assess their performance. In addition, an individual cannot be deemed incompetent if:

● their job description has recently changed
● new systems or technology have been introduced
● they are newly appointed.

These are factors beyond their control and it is your job to ensure appropriate support, training and development are given to meet the appropriate competences or standards.

Other causes of poor performance

If the person's incompetence is due to ill health, you would need to follow the steps outlined in the sickness/absence policy. If it is due to negligence or general unwillingness to carry out duties properly, then it is usually appropriate to follow the disciplinary procedures for misconduct. It's a good idea to check which policy may be more appropriate for the individual situation.

PROCEDURE FOR INCOMPETENCE

Most competence or capability procedures begin with an informal stage where you are required to meet with the member of staff to clarify their role, what is expected and agree a plan with a timetable to achieve the standards. Any training or retraining needs should be established and agreed. Hopefully, with the support of you and your team, the member of staff will improve over the next few weeks/months and no further action will be required.

However, if the problems continue, progression to the formal stage may be indicated. This usually consists of a formal meeting with the member of staff, often with a trade union representative and an HR representative. A further plan with a timetable is then agreed. If it fails again, a further meeting may be agreed with a further plan but this time with a warning that failure to meet the objectives could lead to dismissal.

Throughout the whole process, you need to ensure that you are:

● doing everything you can to encourage improvement
● appreciating the level of improvement attained throughout the process
● identifying and dealing with any extenuating circumstances
● identifying the possibility of moving them to a different ward or department where the skills are better matched to the role
● considering the overall attitude of the employee.

Capability/competency policies vary between organisations. It is wise to ensure you are familiar with your local policy before taking any steps to deal with a member of staff thought to be incompetent in their role.

KNOW WHEN AND HOW TO DISCIPLINE

Never take any action under the disciplinary procedure until you have sought advice from your line manager and HR advisor. It should only be used in extreme cases. Putting a member of your team through the disciplinary process can be very damaging to morale, both for the individual and the rest of the team.

MINOR BREACHES OF CONDUCT

It's better to use a structured meeting or review in cases of minor breaches of conduct or performance. This would constitute an informal discussion, not a disciplinary hearing. It is good practice to make a file note of the conversation and agreed outcomes. Examples of cases that you could deal with on an informal basis include:

- failure to carry out reasonable instructions
- unauthorised absence
- persistent poor time keeping
- poor adherence to the uniform policy.

MAJOR BREACHES OF CONDUCT

The disciplinary policy is one of the few policies where often the first step is to undertake a formal investigation. This is usually undertaken by someone other than the line manager who is not directly involved in the matter. The formal disciplinary procedure may be used for incidents such as:

- physical or verbal assault
- fraud, e.g. falsely claiming unsocial hours payments
- negligent behaviour, which seriously threatens the health and safety of others
- malicious damage
- theft.

Disciplinary action can only be undertaken once a formal investigation of the incident has been carried out. In some cases, police will also need to be involved. Suspension from duty should only be carried out if the person poses a real threat to either patients or staff. Never suspend a member of staff without consulting your senior manager and HR first. Don't be pushed into suspending a member of staff if you feel it is unnecessary. Many NHS workers are left traumatised from unnecessary suspensions (http://www.suspension-nhs.org).

Because the nature of the incident is usually extremely serious, the disciplinary procedure does not consist of a series of meetings like most other policies. It consists of one disciplinary panel, which is brought together to consider the results of the investigation and make a final decision. The panel usually consists of the general manager and an HR representative. Other people present will be the employee, their union representative and, where appropriate, the investigating officer. Witnesses may be required to attend where appropriate. The outcome can be one of the following:

- a verbal warning
- a first written warning
- a final written warning
- a dismissal.

In cases of gross misconduct, the case can also be referred to the Nursing and Midwifery Council (NMC) for further investigation. This may result in the individual's removal from the register.

ACTIVELY MANAGE SICK LEAVE

If your team are well motivated, it is less likely that you will have continual sickness/absence problems. If you do, look first at your leadership style and if there is any way that you can improve your teamwork before dealing with the individual (see Ch. 3).

Most sickness/absence policies clearly lay out the steps that your staff should take when they are sick. This entails phoning you or the nurse-in-charge and informing you of:

- the nature of their illness
- when they expect to return to work
- any work/patient issues that need to be addressed while they are away.

They are usually required to keep in touch at regular intervals and give at least a day's notice before return. You should keep a record of all contacts.

SHORT-TERM SICK LEAVE

Your job is to make sure that all staff who have been off sick are fit for work on their return and to decide if any special arrangements are needed. This means that you (or your deputy) should see every member of staff on return even if only 1 day's sick was taken. You could be liable for any incidents if you allow a member of staff to return and look after vulnerable patients when they are clearly not well enough to do so.

All details should be noted on the person's personnel file. Remember that this is confidential information. As their manager, you are entitled to know about the person's sickness but the rest of the team are not. Keep all staff personal files locked away and do not divulge any information to others.

If the individual does not want you to know the nature of their illness, then it's best to ask your occupational health (OH) department to see them to determine on your behalf that they are fit to return to work.

Take action in cases of continual short episodes of absence

Organisational policies on sickness usually advise a referral to the OH team if staff have more than a certain number of absences over a certain time period; for example, more than three episodes within 6 months.

If you refer to the OH team, make sure that you tell them the reason for referral and what you want to know, otherwise it could be a waste of time.

1. Do you want them to reassure you that the person is now fit for work?
2. Do you want to know if the sickness leave they are taking is reasonable for their condition?
3. Is the sickness liable to continue?
4. If you consider it excessive, ask what is a reasonable level of sickness for their condition?

Check your organisation's sickness/absence policy. It will outline the steps to take if you have a member of staff who continually takes an unacceptably high amount of sickness despite being declared fit for work by the OH department.

What further action can be taken?

The procedure usually starts with a meeting to establish the reasons and set targets. If these are not met, the next step is often a formal meeting. This meeting may result in:

- a further period of monitoring
- a further referral to the OH department
- consideration of a transfer
- a formal caution for a period of around 6 months.

If attendance does not improve, the next stage may lead to a final formal caution for a period of around 12 months. If the behaviour continues after this stage, many policies will then give you the final option of dismissal after a further review.

As a ward manager, you do not have the authority to terminate the employment of your staff. This responsibility lies with your own line manager whom you should fully involve at this stage.

LONG-TERM SICK LEAVE

Long-term sick leave is dealt with very differently. Long-term sick leave is often defined as leave consisting of 4 weeks or more. There is very little you can do when a member of staff has taken long-term sick leave, but you must make sure that the OH department is fully aware and involved.

Whatever the reason, don't forget about someone who is on long-term sick leave. Keep in regular contact. If you cannot keep in contact by letter or phone, you can visit them as long as you have given them prior notice. You are still their manager and therefore should have concern for their welfare.

Don't allow long-term sick leave to affect the rest of your staff

Do not just make do with bank/agency nurses day after day. Can you advertise the post as a secondment for another nurse who wants to gain further experience in your specialty? Can you employ another nurse full time in their place using finances from elsewhere within your directorate? Have you any other vacancies (e.g. health care assistant) from which you can transfer the funding and recruit another nurse? You could also see if it is possible for the person to undertake different duties such as administration, while unable to return to clinical duties for a while. Explore all options involving all departments. Do not cope without that member of staff and let the rest of the team suffer.

Fit for return to work after long-term sick leave?

Always involve the OH department before allowing a member of staff to return to work following long-term sick leave. A decision needs to be made in conjunction with the returning nurse and the OH department as to the terms of their return. They usually have one of four options:

1. Return to the same job as before.
2. Return to the same job but with a graduated return, i.e. part time and then full time.
3. Return to the same ward but with modified duties.
4. Return to a different job, on health grounds.

If the OH team determines that the person will be unable to return to work at all, their employment may be terminated, e.g. retirement on grounds of ill health.

UNAUTHORISED ABSENCE

It is important to take immediate action in any cases of unauthorised absence. If a member of staff does not turn up for work and has made no contact at all, do everything you can to find out where they are. Get someone to physically go around to their home if necessary. Your first major concern is for their welfare. If they are fine, you can deal with it informally depending on the reason. An odd occasion of oversleeping would not warrant formal action, but it would involve a meeting with the person on return.

If you feel they were neglectful, you do have the option of deducting their pay for those days in which they were absent (deducting pay is done by completing a form which you can get from your HR or finance department). In more persistent or major cases of unauthorised absence, the disciplinary procedure may be instigated.

ENSURE ALL STAFF HAVE APPROPRIATE TRAINING, DEVELOPMENT AND SUPPORT

All development needs, including courses and training, should be formally identified through the appraisal process. You only have a certain amount of funding for study days and around 1–2% release time to allocate to your team over the year. Make sure you know exactly what funding you have. You are the budget holder and therefore entitled to have this information.

INDUCTION

Staff induction is the most important teaching package you can have, yet one that is so often neglected. Every new staff member should have the time and opportunity to familiarise themselves with both the organisation and the workings of the ward.

There is no formal requirement as to the length of induction but it would be wise to allocate at least 2 weeks at the beginning, aside from the formal organisational induction, during which the new person is supernumerary. This includes members of staff who are transferred internally. If you can, try to include the mandatory training requirements during this 'supernumerary' induction period. It saves a lot of study leave for the rest of the team for the remaining year.

Following this, you would need some sort of local package detailing the clinical competences that need to be met. All newly qualified staff will need to commence a preceptorship programme and be allocated a preceptor (Department of Health 2010).

WARD-BASED TEACHING

Regular ward-based teaching sessions are a must but don't just think up subjects randomly. Use your regular meetings to assess the learning requirements of your staff. Asking staff what teaching sessions they would like is insufficient on its own. Use your regular reviews of the complaints, incidents and quality indicators to provide information about what your team need. Try to involve the whole team in making such decisions, not the requests of individuals.

A teaching programme devised by one or two members of staff without the full involvement of the rest of the team will not be very motivating. People invited in to teach on the programme may find that few people turn up to their sessions. If staff together identify that they would like more input on a certain subject, they are more likely to prioritise their work during the shift to ensure their attendance.

LEARNING FROM EXPERIENCE

Courses and study days are not the only methods of learning. One of the best ways of learning is through experience. However, without the appropriate support and guidance systems in place, staff will not learn as much as they can from their experiences. Many of us have come across people who have many years of experience but still do not seem to know much or do their job very well.

Your job as the ward manager is to make sure systems are in place so that your staff can gain as much learning from their experience as possible. First, you need to make sure that every member of your team has access to either a preceptor or clinical supervisor. This should be someone who is more experienced than them, but does not necessarily have to be more senior. This more experienced person should be able to work with them or at least meet with them regularly to help them reflect and learn from their day-to-day experiences. If you do not have the skills or capacity within your team to offer this support, try and encourage individual staff to take part in group clinical supervision or an action learning set with other staff of similar grades from other wards.

CLINICAL PRACTICE FACILITATORS

Many hospitals now have staff in the role of clinical practice facilitators who are based in clinical areas and provide support for students and staff as well as providing a vital link with universities. Some cover several wards and departments so it's a good idea to build up a good relationship with your practice facilitator to ensure that your nursing students have a good placement experience, and therefore will want to return to your ward once qualified. The practice facilitators will also support your staff, particularly with students who may need extra assistance to achieve their learning outcomes.

LINK LECTURER

Most wards have a link lecturer from their local university. Work closely with them and identify together how you can best utilise their time. Unless you are proactive and build up a good professional relationship with your link lecturer, you may end up receiving the bare minimum from them. Remember to give something back too. There is no reason why you or your team cannot provide input into work at the university too. The more helpful you are to them, the more helpful they will be in return.

PROVIDE ADDITIONAL SUPPORT FOR MENTORS

Your responsibilities for your team of mentors have been made quite clear (NMC 2006). The only nurses that can formally mentor nursing students are those that have successfully completed an accredited mentor preparation programme, have attended an update within the previous year and are subject to triennial reviews where they need evidence to show that they have mentored at least two students over a 3-year period. All sign-off mentors must have had additional preparation which includes being formally observed signing off students on three separate occasions by a practice teacher or another sign-off mentor. The first two occasions can be simulated (e.g. role play). Your organisation has responsibility for keeping these records and they are checked regularly through NMC visits; however, it's up to you to ensure the records for your area are up-to-date. It is imperative that you do so, especially in cases where you have to deal with appeals from any failing students.

FAILING STUDENTS

The most common reason for failing a student is because of 'attitude' problems (Duffy 2003), as well as problems with competence. In many cases, the problems will begin to show early on in the student's placement, and it's vital that you identify and document them early on too. Don't wait until the mid-way assessment. If the student has a problem, the mentor should raise it with the student and explore the reasons for their behaviour or competence problem. If the student is made aware early on, they have time to work on making improvements with the help of your team of staff. If the student is not made aware early on and your team do not support the student to improve their performance (and have evidence to show that they have done so), then the student has full grounds for appeal. It is advisable to seek support with the documentation from the link lecturer, personal tutor or practice facilitator.

Encourage your staff to give regular feedback to students on their progress. They should encourage the student to assess themselves and acknowledge their concerns. It's always so much easier if students can identify their own problems first rather than be told someone else's point of view. Feedback must always be based on competences (i.e objective) and students should never be compared with others (i.e. subjective). Remember to ensure that the mentors give feedback to their students on what they do well and not to focus only on the negative aspects.

Written evidence always needs to be provided for failing students but it must be based on observation. Mentors must demonstrate that they have observed the student for at least 40% of their placement and sign-off mentors need an additional 1 hour per week of protected time with their student (NMC 2006). It is your duty to ensure that you facilitate this through effective funding and rostering.

MENTOR MEETINGS

Ensure that mentors are given the time and space to meet with their students regularly without interruptions, to discuss their progress. This extra time will have to be planned for within your budget. Do you have funds within your budget to enable mentors to spend time with the nursing students? If not, you should take steps to ensure that it is added (see Ch. 6).

Provide support for your mentors in the form of a regular meeting, preferably each month. This can be facilitated either by you or, better still, by one of the practice facilitators or link lecturer. The mentors should have some sort of forum where they can discuss issues, reflect on their practice and generate ideas for handling various situations.

REDUCE STAFF STRESS

If your staff are stressed at work, it will only serve to increase your problems. Stress in the workplace is a health and safety issue. Organisations are required by law to look at what the risks are and take sensible measures to tackle them (Health and Safety Executive (HSE) 1999). You have certain responsibilities for the health, safety and welfare of your staff. It is important for you to ensure systems are in place to respond to individual concerns. Guidelines are available to help managers meet their legal duties (HSE 2011). These guidelines outline standards that should be met. Your staff should be able to say that:

● they are able to cope with the demands of their job
● they have a say about the way they work
● they receive adequate information from you and their colleagues
● they are not subject to any unacceptable behaviours at work such as bullying

- they understand their roles and responsibilities
- they are engaged frequently when undergoing any organisational change.

Some people are more vulnerable to stress than others, particularly if there are recent changes in their personal circumstances. If allowed to continue, it can affect their health and their performance. It can also affect other members of staff who have to continually cover when their stressed colleagues ring in sick. Ultimately, patient care will suffer.

RECOGNISE THE SIGNS

Be alert to changes in a person's mood or behaviour. They may become quiet and withdrawn, bossy and aggressive or irritable. Their performance at work may be affected. Their standard of work may gradually deteriorate. One obvious sign is increased sickness levels or lateness. Other symptoms often missed are becoming too involved at work, staying behind to make sure things are done or expecting higher and higher standards from self and others.

Look out for the physical symptoms too. These include frequent coughs and colds, headaches, perpetual tiredness and an inability to smile or join in with any banter. The symptoms of stress vary and if you don't know a person well it can be difficult to determine. It is therefore imperative that, as their manager, you make it your business to know all the individuals in your team. You should be familiar with how they think, how they organise themselves and how they work together with the others as a team. A noticeable change in someone's behaviour is the main symptom to be alert to. If you do not know how they behave normally then spotting the changes will be a lot more difficult.

REDUCE THE PRESSURE

Once you have spotted the symptoms of stress, you need to do something about it. The first step is to find out the cause. The only way to find out is to ask, and listen closely to what they have to say. Some common causes of stress in nursing are:

- feeling overloaded
- feeling out of one's depth
- feeling undervalued
- feeling alone and unsupported
- lacking confidence
- being uncertain about the future, the role or work environment
- pressures from home such as childcare or money worries
- being bullied or harassed.

If any of your staff say they feel overloaded, out of their depth, undervalued or alone, then they need extra support. You can do this yourself or it may be more appropriate to assign one of the more senior and experienced people in your team to do this.

Giving support is more than just spending time listening and giving advice. On its own, this solves little. Support involves taking practical action too. If the problem is work overload or feeling out of depth, try working closely with them for a few shifts, observing how they manage their time and helping them to improve any skills deficit. If the problem is feeling undervalued or a lack of confidence, try increasing feedback (both positive and negative) on their day-to-day performance. Consistent feedback helps by showing them what they do right and what they need to do to improve. It helps individuals to take control of their work and feel that they are making progress.

If members of your staff are stressed due to uncertainty about changes at work, this may indicate that you have not involved them enough in the process of change. You may have kept them informed, but there is a huge difference between informing and involving staff. Make sure they feel their opinions are heard and acted upon.

If someone has pressures at home causing undue stress at work, you are not obliged to sort out their home circumstances but consider what you can do to help at work. Possible solutions may include allowing them a short period of leave or a change in working hours.

If any members of your staff are being bullied or harassed, take action to stop it now. Give them some time out from the situation or move staff if necessary. Involve human resources (HR) straight away for advice and support on the best approach to follow. Never leave a situation like this to solve itself (see p. 251).

INFORM AND INVOLVE ALL OF YOUR TEAM

If people are given a say about the way they do their work, receive adequate information and support, and are fully engaged in any organisational changes, they are more likely to maintain high levels of health, wellbeing and performance (HSE 2011). In other words, you will have fewer problems with sickness absence, high staff turnover and poor performance.

Be completely open and honest with your team about everything that is going on. Generally the only information that you need to keep confidential is the personal details of your staff members. Question any manager that says 'don't tell your staff until we say so'. Unless it involves private and personal staff details, nothing should be confidential.

INFORMATION FROM MEETINGS

When you attend the meetings held by your line manager or nursing director, let your staff know of all decisions that have been made and any information you have gained. Just giving your staff the minutes to read through is generally insufficient. They do not know which bits are important and may not understand or have time to read through the jargon. Highlight the parts that are pertinent to them. Clarify for them what the decisions mean.

INVOLVEMENT IN MAKING DECISIONS

Keeping staff informed about everything to do with the ward is essential, but even more important is getting them involved. Be honest. If you are unsure how a future change is going to affect their jobs then say so, but make sure you involve them in the process of finding out.

Try not to make all managerial decisions by yourself. Involve your team. If, for example, you involve them in managing your budget and the roster, they will understand the importance of ensuring that everyone books their annual leave in advance and therefore will be more likely to do so.

BUSINESS PLANNING AND RECRUITMENT

Involve your team in the business planning process each year and in monitoring how the budget is being spent.

Review your budget statement with your team each month. When a member of staff leaves, review with your team what the role should be and what should be put in the advert. Identify who wants to be involved in the interviews and whether the selection process should involve a presentation. This is a far better way of treating your staff than just informing them that your budget is overspent or you are recruiting another member of staff.

PLANNING THE TEAM'S STUDY LEAVE

When deciding each year how to allocate your study leave for the team, involve them in that decision too. List all the courses that staff would like to undertake in the coming year. Add up all the study days these will cost the team. Let them know how many study days you have to allocate over the year (usually around 1–2% of your budget, see p. 109) and decide between you who and what take priority.

Your staff will be far more motivated if they can see the restrictions to which you are working. Understanding why the decision needs to be made leaves them a lot less willing to find someone to blame if they cannot have all the study leave they would like.

INVESTIGATING COMPLAINTS

Investigating and writing a response to a complainant is an excellent learning experience, not only for the person you delegate the investigation to, but also for the whole team. Share the results of the investigation and the difficulties you had during the process. Show them the final response letter and ask if they all agree with what you are saying. This not only gives them an insight into the problem, it keeps them involved. It shows that you truly value your team and their opinions.

CONSIDER TEAM-BASED SELF-ROSTERING

By having shared goals and an action plan, you are well on the way to ensuring your staff work better together. Getting them to appreciate each others' needs is another hurdle. One way you can do this is through team-based self-rostering. Self-rostering does not mean having everyone writing down when they want to work and whoever gets there last gets the worst shift pattern! It also does not mean having everyone fill in their requests on a draft roster. Self-rostering is about giving your staff the flexibility to cover the shifts in their team in their own way instead of your way.

SELF-ROSTERING IS EASIER IN SMALL TEAMS

Don't implement self-rostering for the whole team to do at once. There is no way you can get them all together for a start. There are far too many of them and you cannot leave the ward without cover. The ideal way to self-roster is within teams.

Many wards nowadays are divided into two or three teams. Give each team their part of the roster and ask them to sort it out among themselves to cover their patients on a 24-hour basis. They will soon become more aware of each others' needs and more willing to give and take. They will be more aware about who needs to work with their mentor and who needs time off to take their children to football practice every Thursday evening, for example. They will have to decide among themselves who is more deserving of having certain weekends off. They will have to choose between the one who wants to go to the wedding or the one who wants to go to a concert. Leaving it for your staff to decide among themselves in small teams makes them appreciate each others' needs far better than if the decision was left to you.

If you are restricted to having one senior staff nurse on per shift from either team, it may be easier to get one team to do their part of the roster first, then the next team to devise their part around it. They can swap over next time to make the process fair. It ensures that there is always an appropriate senior member in charge per shift.

The Department of Health produced some handy guidelines for team-based self-rostering in 2003. Although these have not been updated since, they are worth a perusal (Department of Health 2003).

ADVANTAGES OF SELF-ROSTERING

There are many advantages to team-based self-rostering. The benefits for staff include:

- having more control over their working lives
- linking start and finish times to travel restrictions
- covering for each other to fit in with family care arrangements
- opting for fewer longer shifts or shorter split shifts to cover for each other
- more control to be at work for individual work commitments, e.g. link nurse meetings or patient case conferences
- more control in planning team activity.

SET ROSTERS WITH SET LINES

Another option of giving staff more autonomy in their shift pattern is to have a master roster. This is where each member of staff has a set line within the roster. You can then give your staff the option of swapping lines or individual shifts between themselves to meet their personal requirements. This is less flexible but could be a good starting point rather than going for complete self-rostering straight away.

ACTION POINTS

- Arrange regular monthly meetings with your HR advisor to discuss any day-to-day problems or potential problems and to keep each other up-to-date.
- Start keeping brief file notes of day-to-day meetings and phone conversations.
- Set up a communication book/folder for staff if you do not have one already.
- Delegate appraisals to staff, ensuring they have the appropriate skills to do so, and make appointments in your diary for those you need to do yourself.
- Read through and familiarise yourself with your sickness/absence policy, competence/capability policy and disciplinary policy.
- Make sure you see every member of staff on return from sick leave and make a brief file note if you don't already do so.
- Set dates for monthly staff meetings to review the budget, complaints, serious incidents, etc., and involve your team in any decisions.
- Set up an induction package for all new staff (include all mandatory sessions for the year), and review ongoing teaching packages with your team.
- Set up a regular meeting for your team of mentors to reflect and discuss issues with mentoring students. This can be facilitated by yourself, the practice facilitator or link lecturer.
- Make sure any members of your staff displaying any signs of stress are managed appropriately.

References

Department of Health, 2003. Working lives: programmes for change: team-based self-rostering. DH Publications, London. Online. Available: http://www.dh.gov.uk/assetRoot/04/03/50/32/04035032.pdf Jan 2012.

Department of Health, 2010. Preceptorship framework for newly registered nurses, midwives and allied health professionals. CNO Directorate, London.

Duffy, K., 2003. Failing students: a qualitative study of factors that influence the decisions regarding the assessment of students' competence in practice. NMC, London. Online. Available: http://www.nmc-uk.org/Documents/Archived%20Publications/1Research%20 papers/Kathleen_Duffy_Failing_Students2003.pdf Jan 2012.

Health and Safety Executive, 1999. The management of health and safety at work regulations. Online. Available: http://www.legislation.gov.uk/uksi/1999/3242/contents/made Jan 2012.

Health and Safety Executive, 2011. What are the management standards for work-related stress? HSE, Suffolk. Online. Available: http://www.hse.gov.uk/stress/standards/index.htm Jan 2012.

Information Commissioner, 1998. The Data Protection Act. HMSO, London. Online. Available: http://www.informationcommissioner.gov.uk Jan 2012.

Nursing and Midwifery Council, 2006. Standards to support learning and assessment in practice. NMC, London. Online. Available: http://www.nmc-uk.org/Documents/Standards/nmcStandardsToSupportLearningAndAssessmentInPractice.pdf Jan 2012.

The NHS Staff Council, 2010. Appraisals and KSF made simple – a practical guide. Online. Available: http://www.nhsemployers.org/Aboutus/Publications/Documents/Appraisals%20and%20KSF%20made%20simple.pdf Jan 2012.

MAKE SURE CARE IS PATIENT-CENTRED

Many ward managers will say that the care they provide on their ward is patient-centred, but is it really? If your team still undertake drug rounds at set times or carry out observations at set times, then the care is not patient-centred. It is centred around staff routine. Truly patient-centred care means that care is centred around the patient's needs, not the staff's needs or ward routines.

The only way you can provide truly patient-centred care is to ensure that there are systems and processes in place to find out what your patients really need and then to base your care around those needs. This chapter takes a look at those systems and processes required to maintain a high standard of patient-centred care.

MAINTAIN YOUR CLINICAL SKILLS

Keeping up-to-date clinically is essential for the ward manager role. You cannot maintain high standards of care without having a thorough knowledge of your specialty. You need an in-depth knowledge of your subject to be able to act as a role model for others. You may also need to protect the patients from others who are less experienced, including junior doctors, and 'performance-indicator'-orientated managers.

Having defined your workload (see Ch. 2), you may find that you can spend only four half-days a week on the ward in a clinical capacity, so you should make the most of this time.

ACCESSING UP-TO-DATE INFORMATION

Make sure you have full access to appropriate up-to-date textbooks on your specialty. Keep them in your office for you and your staff to refer to when necessary. You can source funding for textbooks through:

- your stationery budget
- ward funds
- one of the hospital charities, e.g. League of Friends.

You should have full access to professional journals through the NHS library. The NHS Evidence Web site is accessible to all: http://www.evidence.nhs.uk. Plus, you should have full access to the following:

- NHS Athens if you work in England: http://www.openathens.net
- Health on the Net in Northern Ireland (honni): http://www.honni.qub.ac.uk
- The Knowledge Network for those in Scotland: http://www.knowledge.scot.nhs.uk/home.aspx
- NHS Wales e-Library for Health: http://www.wales.nhs.uk/sitesplus/878.

In addition, you should be regularly accessing all sites which offer evidence-based clinical guidelines such as those produced by the National Institute for Health and Clinical Excellence for England and Wales: http://www.nice.org.uk and the Scottish Intercollegiate Guidelines Network: http://www.sign.ac.uk.

Print off any pertinent articles/relevant research and leave copies on the coffee table in the staff room. It's a simple way of enabling both yourself and your staff to keep up-to-date.

CLINICAL SUPERVISION

Having an appropriate clinical supervisor is essential for you to help maintain your professional competence and credibility. Find someone who is more experienced and expert than you. One of the senior consultants (nurse or doctor) linked with your ward is a good option. Another more experienced ward manager or perhaps the link lecturer may be suitable. Meet with them regularly to reflect and learn from your experiences. Regular clinical supervision will enable you to:

- stop picking up bad habits
- challenge yourself and think more deeply about certain areas of practice
- get advice and support.

If you cannot find anyone more experienced than you, then the next best option is to set up a group of people and meet once per month to reflect on practice together (see p. 177).

LEARNING THROUGH TEACHING OTHERS

Invite staff or student nurses to shadow you regularly for a shift. This not only gives them valuable experience but their enquiring minds will help stimulate your thinking and question your practice. Giving regular teaching sessions also keeps you 'on the ball'. Teaching is a valuable learning experience for the teacher as well as the student. And if you find you are unable to answer any questions, go and find out the answer together.

ENSURE THAT ALL PATIENTS HAVE A FULL ASSESSMENT AND CARE PLAN

Care planning is an essential part of patient care, but in times of staffing shortages or increased workload it becomes low on the priority list for some. Yet without a specific document outlining the plan of care, important issues are likely to be missed. Care planning provides a guide to all who are involved with the patient's care, including temporary staff.

It is essential that all patients are fully assessed using an appropriate nursing model, not a tick sheet. The written plan of care should be based on that assessment. This may seem basic but it's still known for some patients to be discharged without having had a nursing assessment or written plan of care throughout their hospital stay.

Care plans save so much time, particularly if you have to use bank and agency nurses regularly. They ensure handovers are safe and efficient. Staff do not have to keep explaining what needs to be done for the patient if it's written in the care plan. Bank and agency nurses don't have to keep interrupting other staff during the course of their shift to ask questions about their patients' care.

If a patient does not have a care plan, nurses have little defence against allegations of negligence. Legally, it will be assumed that the nursing care was not planned if there is no evidence of a care plan.

WHICH MODEL?

Roper, Logan and Tierney's model of nursing still appears to be the most popular method in the UK as it incorporates all activities of daily living. Orem's self-care deficit model and the Neuman systems model are still in use in some areas. More recent models being introduced include the Gloucester Patient Profile, which focuses solely on physical aspects of care. It is becoming more popular because of its usefulness in auditing and as a trigger tool (Thompson and Wright 2003).

It's entirely up to you and your team which model you use; just make sure that you choose one that is relevant to your patients' needs, and don't be 'brow-beaten' into replacing it by paperwork based on 'performance indicators' only. (For a good overview of nursing models in practice, read Barrett et al 2009.) You must have some sort of nursing assessment system in place that identifies the patients' nursing requirements, followed by a written plan of care.

STANDARDISED CARE PLANS

Standardised care plans save time but try to ensure that your team adapt them to an individual patient's needs. Sometimes with standardised care plans, people can get used to seeing the same old thing. As a result, you may find that they tend not to read or refer to them. If you specify to your team that they must write the patients' individual needs on the care plan in addition to the routine predicted needs, it will increase the likelihood of them being read.

Some nurses are under the misconception that writing the patient's name under each problem heading is individualising the standardised care plan. This is unnecessary and serves no useful purpose other than to waste precious time. The patient's name only has to be written once on each sheet of paper.

ACCOUNTABILITY

As the ward manager, you are responsible for ensuring the *systems* are in place to ensure that every single patient in your ward receives a full nursing assessment and care plan. The registered nurses in your team are responsible for the *content* of the assessment, care plan and subsequent evaluations. The Nursing and Midwifery Council (NMC) code clearly states for nurses that: 'You must keep clear and accurate records of the discussions you have, the assessments you make, the treatment and medicines you give and how effective these have been' (NMC 2008).

Get your team together and use their skills and experience to decide on which model is the most appropriate for assessing and planning care for the type of patients you have on your ward. If they have taken part in choosing which model to use, they are more likely to be willing to use that model in their day-to-day practice.

CARE PLANS AS TEACHING TOOLS

Make sure your staff write clear care plans. The goals and actions should be specific and measurable. For example, a goal for a post-surgical patient such as 'to prevent a chest infection' is not specific. A goal such as 'to remain free from chest infection as evidenced by T < 37 °C, WBC between 4–11, lungs clear on auscultation and negative sputum culture' is a lot more meaningful. When care plans are used this way, they can also be invaluable teaching tools.

CARE PLANS AS COMMUNICATION TOOLS

The ultimate purpose of care plans is to inform everyone in the team of the patients' care needs. Any nurse coming back from 'days off' or annual leave and unfamiliar with the patient should be able to find all the information they need in the care plan. If there is no care plan, they will waste time trying to find out.

To condone the non-use of care plans on your ward equates to allowing poor standards of communication and patient care. Lack of care plans increases the risk of untoward incidents and unintentional neglect. Around 10% of NMC hearings concerning fitness to practise are due to allegations of 'failure to maintain accurate records' (NMC 2011), which includes the lack of care plans.

BE CLEAR ABOUT WHAT HEALTH CARE ASSISTANTS CAN AND CANNOT DO

The role of the health care assistant (HCA) in supporting registered nurses has always been a contentious issue. The main concern is usually around the nurses' accountability for the actions of HCAs. The NMC code states clearly that it is up to the individual nurse delegating the task to decide in each situation whether the HCA has the appropriate skills and competence (NMC 2008):

- You must establish that anyone you delegate to is able to carry out your instructions.
- You must confirm that the outcome of any delegated task meets required standards.
- You must make sure that everyone you are responsible for is supervised and supported.

HCAs are as much a part of the team as registered nurses. Unfortunately, there are some managers who insist on having separate handovers for registered staff, and some that don't include HCAs in the handover process at all. Handovers must include the whole team. The registered nurses and HCAs can then plan the care of their patients together.

GIVE HCAs RESPONSIBILITY, NOT TASKS

Delegating tasks creates a 'them and us' atmosphere. With the emphasis on
achieving competencies for diploma (equivalent to NVQ) levels 2, 3 and 4, HCAs
are becoming more highly skilled. Rather than delegate a series of tasks to HCAs, it
is more appropriate to delegate a small case load of patients with supervision. This
maximises the use of their skills and abilities by enabling them to carry out the care
as prescribed in the care plans. It enables HCAs to use their initiative rather than
complete a set of delegated tasks. The registered nurses remain available to assist in
areas where the HCAs do not have the competence to carry out a nursing task.

HCAs should also be included in all team and decision-making processes. At
the time of writing this book, HCAs are not a regulated profession although in
Scotland they are required to comply with the HCA code of conduct, which is
regulated through their employing organisation (NHS Scotland 2011). Given
the current trend towards reducing the number of registered nurses while
correspondingly increasing the reliance on HCAs, it is likely that some form of
regulation will be introduced across the UK in the future, even if it is simply a code
of conduct that is implemented at organisational level. In the meantime, if the
registered nurse has ensured that care is delegated according to the specifications
of the NMC code as outlined previously, the HCA is then accountable for the care
(RCN 2008).

HCA TRAINING AND DEVELOPMENT

It is your role as the ward manager to ensure that HCAs have the appropriate
training, are assessed as competent and are confident in their own ability to care for
patients and perform certain tasks. You must keep records of all training attended
and assessments undertaken and ensure that clear guidelines and protocols are in
place. It is also advisable that you are familiar with the assessment, training and
competences required for each diploma level (levels 2 and 3 enable HCAs to take
responsibility for the care of a group of patients whose care plans have already been
written by a registered nurse).

Review the HCA job description regularly and ensure it acknowledges any
additional responsibilities. The job description should also clearly state the role
boundaries.

ELIMINATE LONG HANDOVERS

If handovers are continually taking much more than half an hour, then perhaps you
and your team need to revise the way they are carried out. Precious time for patient
care is being lost. Long handovers cause resentment among those hanging around
waiting for a well-earned break or to go home.

The shift handover is a crucial period for maintaining communication and
continuity of care. The importance of getting the system right should not be
underestimated.

OFFICE HANDOVERS

Advantages

Office handovers can be quick and effective if carried out properly without devolving into lengthy discussions about each patient. They avoid the risk of being continually interrupted by visitors, other health professionals or the patients themselves. There is also minimal risk of other patients and visitors overhearing confidential details.

Disadvantages

The problem with office handovers is that the patient is not involved at all. The handover may not always be based on the plan of care, which stays by the patient's bedside. When shut away in the office, the reporting nurse may become judgemental, giving the next shift's nurses preconceived ideas about the patients they are about to care for. In addition, office handovers used alone can become very lengthy, especially if the nurse who does the first few patients then has to go and find the relevant nurse to hand over the next few patients and so on.

BEDSIDE HANDOVERS

Advantages

Bedside handovers allow for greater patient involvement. Patients have the opportunity to contribute. The nurse taking over for the next shift can put a face to the name and remember more easily who is who without having to resort to the piece of paper in their pocket. It also negates the need for the nurses to visit all the patients after handover to introduce themselves and familiarise themselves with their care plans.

Disadvantages

The problem with bedside handovers is that in some areas they have devolved from a 'bedside' handover to an 'end of bed' handover. This rather impersonal approach is similar to some doctors' rounds where the patient care is discussed between health professionals without the participation of the patient. The only patient involvement is through unavoidable eavesdropping. It can also be difficult to maintain patient confidentiality with 'end of bed' handovers.

COMBINATION HANDOVERS

A combination of office handover based on 'name, age and diagnosis' followed by a bedside handover using the care plans can be the most efficient and effective process of handing over between shifts. The first part in the office should be kept brief. The receiving nurses would then divide up into teams to receive a full handover by the patients' beds, but only for the patients they will be looking after. This keeps the handover focused and relevant. It maintains the advantages of each method and reduces the disadvantages.

Ways of reducing the length of handover include:

- handing out printed versions with the patient's name and bed number to each nurse coming on duty
- using taped handovers
- ensuring the handover is based on the patient's care plan
- nurses to only receive detailed handover for the group of patients they have been allocated to care for
- having a system of allocating nurses to patients to ensure that, as far as possible, the same staff care for the same patients each shift.

There have been some studies and general debate about the effectiveness of non-verbal and taped handovers but beware of using these methods as the only means of handover. A report produced by the Health and Safety Executive into effective shift handover studied five major disasters (including the Piper Alpha disaster) which were caused by faults in the shift handover system (Lardner 1996). The report concluded that effective shift handovers should always:

- be conducted face-to-face
- be two-way, with both participants taking joint responsibility for ensuring accurate communication
- use verbal and written means of communication
- be given as much time as necessary to ensure accurate communication.

CONFIDENTIALITY AND BEDSIDE HANDOVERS

Make sure that your team maintain confidentiality when handing over their patients by the bedside. The nurses should preferably sit down with the patient and discuss the care plan together. This helps to prevent others overhearing. If the patient has visitors, the handover can be carried out quietly and confidentially between the team elsewhere.

It is advisable not to leave the care plans at the end of the patients' beds for anyone, including visitors, to pick up and read. Leave them *with* the patient at the head of the bed or in their bedside locker. If the patient is confused, or unable to look after their care plan for some other reason such as post-surgery, the care plan should be kept somewhere safe such as by the nurses' station.

In addition, you must have some sort of system for your team to dispose of their handover notes at the end of the shift. Order a confidentiality waste bin or a shredder from your stationery budget and put it somewhere prominent in the staff coffee/changing room.

USE TASK-ORIENTATED CARE ONLY WHEN APPROPRIATE

Many nurses say their chosen method of nursing care delivery is patient allocation, team nursing or primary nursing. Few would admit to carrying out task-orientated care. Yet in reality this is what is happening in many areas. Take the expression,

'You do the "obs" and I'll do the drugs'. Does that sound familiar? It is so easy to fall back into task allocation without realising it is happening. Task allocation is sometimes necessary if the workload increases unexpectedly or in times of acute nursing shortage. If it is a shared decision, there is no problem with this approach. It can be necessary in times of severe nursing shortages.

In fact, with the increasing strain on staffing levels, methods of task allocation are currently being introduced formally such as 'hourly rounding'. If patient-centred care is not working due to reduced staffing levels (evidenced by increased numbers of incidents and complaints), then sometimes task allocation is no bad thing in order to maintain patient safety.

DELEGATION OF CARE

Whatever model of nursing care delivery you use, the overall responsibility for the patient's care should be assigned to registered nurses only. However, apart from giving out medications, HCAs who are trained to diploma (or old NVQ) level 2 or level 3 standard are usually competent to implement most of the care that a nurse can. As long as the patients have clear and up-to-date care plans, there is no reason why HCAs cannot be allocated the care of patients under the supervision of a registered nurse. They can make their own decisions as to what gets done and when. It's much better than being allocated tasks. Resorting to task allocation over long periods of time tends to induce apathy and reduce team morale.

DELEGATION OF TASKS

If you have HCAs who have not attained their diploma (or NVQ equivalent) qualification and the associated competences, task allocation may be the most suitable way of allocating the workload. After all, the registered nurses are ultimately accountable for patient care. However, if you do not give your HCAs the opportunity to develop through the diploma system, you are preventing them from taking on additional responsibilities, resulting in unnecessarily high workloads for your registered nurses.

TASK ALLOCATION IS INCOMPATIBLE WITH THE NURSING PROCESS

Although task allocation can be deemed appropriate in some circumstances (i.e. in times of staffing shortages), it is better to aim for a more patient-centred delivery system. The emphasis on tasks removes the notion of individualised patient care. It is therefore incompatible with the nursing process. This probably explains why in some areas it is considered unimportant for patients to have care plans. If the patients do not have care plans and care is centred on achieving tasks, the bulk of the responsibility lies with one person; the nurse-in-charge. This is not an ideal situation. Working towards a team or 'named nurse' approach (or primary nursing) is a much fairer system for all your staff and a more satisfying way of working.

WORK TOWARDS THE NAMED NURSE (OR PRIMARY NURSING)

To be able to admit a patient, plan their care and look after them every time you are on duty through to their discharge is a very satisfying experience. People take pride in their work. The named nurse does not necessarily have to care for their own patients during their shift. They can delegate to other nurses or HCAs, who can also care for the patient when they are on 'days off'. The named nurse carries responsibility for writing the care plan and ensuring that long-term goals are met, rather than just the short-term goals during the span of one shift.

PATIENT ALLOCATION

The main problem with patient allocation is that nobody takes responsibility for the whole patient care package. Who is responsible if a patient's discharge was not planned and implemented effectively during their stay? Who is responsible if a patient's condition deteriorated over 3 days and nothing was done? If nurses care for a group of patients on one shift, then another group on the next shift, they will not only have less responsibility but also less pride in a job done well.

TEAM NURSING

In theory, team nursing is better than patient allocation. The team leader is the person who takes responsibility for each patient in the team from admission through to discharge. In practice, this does not always happen. Some wards simply split the number of beds into two or three groups and allocate a team of nurses to each area. Each team leader than allocates patients to the team members after handover. It then becomes patient allocation but within smaller teams. However, team nursing can help in areas where there are fewer registered nurses.

NAMED NURSE/PRIMARY NURSING

In theory, named nursing sounds perfect, but when you are 'running on bank and agency' almost every shift, it is not always feasible. However, each named nurse would have other nurses who care for the patient in their absence. It is something that could be quite difficult to organise on a roster when you do not have your full staffing establishment, but once you do, it can work very well.

THE BEST METHOD OF CARE FOR YOUR WARD

A simpler way to ensure nurses take more responsibility is to establish a form of named nursing based on the organisation of care that you already have in place in your ward. You just need to establish a system whereby the nurse who undertakes the initial patient assessment and care plan will be the patient's main nurse throughout their stay. If they are coming up for 'days off', it's up to them to ensure that another nurse will take on that responsibility for the next few days instead. The named nurse does not necessarily have to be allocated the patient to care for on every shift (although it is the ideal option). They just need to be the 'named nurse' responsible for ensuring the patient receives the appropriate care, by regularly reviewing the care plan and delegating as necessary.

Accept that the system will not be perfect and you will not be able to ensure it is fully implemented for every single patient who comes to your ward. Fluctuating staffing levels, increased patient turnover and the continual moving of patients from one ward to another make it extremely difficult to run any model of nursing care delivery effectively. The best you can do is to aim for your patients to be content in the knowledge that there is a specific individual who is responsible for their care from admission to discharge.

MAKE SURE PATIENTS ARE INFORMED

The NMC code states clearly that: 'You must act as an advocate for those in your care, helping them to access relevant health and social care, information and support' (NMC 2008). In addition, you should ensure the provision of sufficient details about the care, treatment and support options so that patients can make an informed decision (Care Quality Commission (CQC) 2010). As a manager, there are three good systems you can introduce to keep the patient and their relatives informed (and prevent your staff being continually interrupted for basic information):

1. A 'welcome' information board.
2. An information board for comments and suggestions.
3. Information sheets and leaflets.

A 'WELCOME' INFORMATION BOARD

Put up a board near the entrance to your ward, to inform new patients and relatives when they first come to be admitted or visit. Some suggestions include:

- a welcome sentence in large print
- directions on where to go and who to report to
- a photograph and information on who the ward manager is and their role
- a photograph and information on who the matron is, their role and contact details
- an explanation about who is who and how to identify staff by their uniforms
- which team or individual staff are looking after which bed numbers (no patient names because of confidentiality)
- the ward layout, including the bed numbers and where they can find the toilets (including directions for visitors' toilets)
- a sentence asking if there is any further information currently not up on the board which they would like to see.

AN INFORMATION BOARD FOR COMMENTS AND SUGGESTIONS

Most wards and departments now have suggestions boxes but many say they are rarely used or leave it to another department to pick up the comments cards. I would suggest this is something that you keep control of with your team. Encourage patients and relatives to use it by putting extracts of their comments up on the board (removing any names and confidential information) accompanied by a written response. Renew them each month. This may help prevent your staff being hassled for things. If, for example, one of the bathrooms is out of action, you can put up a written response on the board saying that the estates department are aware but there are problems with the plumbing that will take around 2 weeks to fix. This will stop patients and relatives continually complaining to your staff.

When you first put up the board, you will probably get very few or no suggestions. One idea to start the process would be to put up some examples. If, for example, you are continually being asked about the short visiting times, write up a response to a sample comment card explaining why you have had to restrict the visiting times. Magazines use a similar approach to attract people to read about certain issues. People are more likely to read a problem page than read an article on the subject.

INFORMATION SHEETS AND LEAFLETS

Ensure you have as much written information as you can readily available for patients. Coming into hospital is such an overwhelming experience for some that they rarely take in half that is being said.

First, ensure that there is some sort of leaflet or information sheet for when they arrive onto your ward which explains things like what the different uniforms mean and where to get a cup of tea. Many hospitals provide this information in leaflet form. If yours does not, it would not take long to compile your own local one. Second, make sure patients have a leaflet explaining their condition or the investigations or surgery they have come in for. It's advisable not to devise leaflets of your own without first looking up to see if there are any other sources you can tap into. There are many good Web sites that produce information leaflets, which you can download or adapt for your own area, such as the following:

- http://www.patient.co.uk: This has over 900 leaflets on health and disease, including tests and investigations.
- http://www.medinfo.co.uk: This site provides information sheets for patients on common conditions and drugs.
- http://www.cks.nhs.uk: This site is aimed at health care professionals providing advice, information and useful links as well as downloadable patient information leaflets.
- http://www.pharmweb.net: This site contains useful links to various specialist Web sites about drugs and conditions.

Producing your own information for patients and relatives

If you wish to produce your own patient information sheets or leaflets within
the NHS, there are specific guidelines which you must adhere to regarding the
presentation and the need for the appropriate logo and colour. The NHS brand
guidelines give guidance on how to devise written information leaflets and
provide templates to help you, including access to a downloadable NHS logo
(NHS 2012).

The main things to remember when writing your information sheets or leaflets
are the following:

1. Present all information in at least 12 point font, preferably bigger.
2. Try not to use words of more than two syllables.
3. Keep the sentences to no more than 15–20 words long.
4. Make it personal by using 'we' and 'you'.
5. Explain any instructions, e.g. if you tell someone not to drive for 2 weeks after
   the operation, explain why.
6. A question and answer format tends to be more favoured by patients.
7. Cover only one investigation or condition per leaflet.
8. Encourage your staff to write the patient's name on the information sheet as it
   will make them more likely to read it.

Never produce patient information without having it endorsed by your
organisation. If you do, you could become personally liable for the information
given, particularly with regards to clinical advice. Most organisations have
some sort of central committee which oversees all patient information produced
internally. You should also ensure that all clinicians (including the consultants)
involved in the specialism have had the opportunity to view and comment on
the leaflet/information sheet before submitting it to your organisation's patient
information group for ratification.

PERFORMANCE INDICATORS, AUDITS AND BENCHMARKING

FOCUS ON CARE, NOT PAPERWORK

Given the trend towards an ever-reducing number of nurses per patient, it is
not really surprising that certain standards of care are perhaps not as good as
they could be. But using an audit or benchmarking tool to confirm these poor
standards is not hugely helpful on its own. (For advice on increasing staff, see
Ch. 6.) Having to undertake audits can just add to the ever-increasing workload.
We all groan whenever auditing, benchmarking or performance indicators
are mentioned, but most of the standards are simply common sense and it's a
sad reflection on our current care provision that such tools are needed at all.
However, they cannot be ignored and you have to ensure that standards on your
ward measure up to standards throughout your organisation. Just make sure
that you focus on making the identified improvements rather than filling in the
paperwork.

Do not deprive your patients of nursing care in order to take part in audit work. If it comes to a choice between patient care and filling in an audit form, patient care must take priority; the audit figures can wait if that is the case. Patient safety is paramount. Mid Staffordshire NHS Trust achieved their 4-hour waiting targets in 2007 but to what cost? Later reports have shown that the focus on these targets (and thus reducing costs) was partly responsible for their higher than average mortality figures (Healthcare Commission 2009). Don't allow your performance indicator monitoring to take priority over actual patient care.

USE AUDIT TOOLS WISELY

If you are asked to audit an aspect of care, don't do it immediately unless you have something to gain from the results. Your team are there to provide care, not to spend their time filling in audit forms. At the time of writing, there are a plethora of performance indicators being monitored. In England, as well as having to meet the Essential Standards of Quality and Safety (CQC 2010) and the eight High Impact Actions, you have further nursing indicators that your trust has agreed to meet in order to meet targets from the commissioning groups. This all takes time. Estimate how much time you need to audit (for example, how many hours per month you spend filling in forms showing the numbers of patients with infections, pressure ulcers or having suffered a fall) and get these hours put into your budget in terms of nurses, or even a part-time administrator perhaps.

In addition, if you are asked to undertake a new audit as part of a project (national or local), don't take it on without the funding to do so or agree which of the current projects you are working on you are willing to 'drop' in order for you and your staff to devote time to this new audit.

BENCHMARKING

Benchmarking takes the process of auditing one step further. It's a process of comparing audits from different areas. The idea is that all areas make improvements to attain the same standards as the one that had the best audit results. The Essence of Care benchmarking tool in England is one example and comprises 12 aspects of care. Each of these is made up of a range of factors. The idea is that you and your team get together to choose an aspect of care that is relevant to your ward and then assess your work against these factors. You decide between you what you think indicates best practice. Once you have done this, you can get together with other wards and departments and compare each others' results. Those who marked themselves high can share any good practice. Those who marked themselves low can take action to improve their own service to match those departments at the higher level. The meetings can stimulate debate as to what constitutes best practice and evidence will need to be produced. The toolkit gives statements and ideas to stimulate your thinking. Again, you will need to ensure that you have funding within your budget to enable you or your staff to undertake the audits and attend the benchmark meetings.

MANAGE STAFFING SHORTAGES

Nurses have an amazing ability to cope when short-staffed. The trouble is just that – they cope. And it's tiring work covering for absent staff as well as your own workload day after day. It can only lead to exhaustion and increased sickness levels, which just serves to make matters worse. It will not come as a surprise to learn that 80% of us have reported increased workloads and are struggling with staff shortages (UNISON 2009).

In the long term, your role is to ensure your staffing levels match the workload through:

- effective rostering (including study and annual leave)
- being fully involved in the business planning process, so that you have the appropriate number of staff required for the workload
- taking extra initiatives to recruit and retain staff
- managing staff sickness.

However, there will be shifts when you have staff sickness, vacancies or unexpected increases in workload and are unable to 'fill' with bank or agency staff. Carrying on and coping on these shifts is still unacceptable.

STOP COPING

When a shift is short of staff and/or the workload for that day has increased unexpectedly, some adopt the attitude that the team have no other option but to just cope and get on with it. This is not appropriate and an example of poor leadership. Good leadership is ensuring that the team spends time at the beginning of the shift making conscious decisions about work that will be left undone as well as planning and prioritising the work that needs to be done. For example, if you have two staff down on an early shift (and there are no bank or agency staff available), the rest of the team should not try to get all the work done and resign to accepting incidents where care is substandard. Phrases such as, 'It can't be helped, we were short-staffed' or 'I didn't get round to doing that because it was so short-staffed this morning' are not acceptable. Poor staffing is not an excuse for poor care.

PRIORITISE – HIGH STANDARDS OF CARE OR SAFETY?

When your team have exhausted all other avenues of getting staff, they must sit down and prioritise. At times like these, you still have to assert some control over your workload. Get your team to decide together at the beginning of the shift what they absolutely must do to maintain the safety of all patients. Then identify together the following:

- Which aspects of care are essential for safety, e.g. food and fluids, medications, constant observation.

- Which aspects of care can be done to a lesser standard or not done at all, e.g. hygiene, rehabilitation activities, information giving.
- Which aspects can be left undone until the next shift or next day, e.g. complex discharges, certain wound dressings, rehabilitation activities, further admissions, any paperwork that does not directly relate to patient care.

These decisions should be made together, documented and the appropriate line manager informed at the beginning of the shift. Don't allow the decision to remain at ward level. The rest of your organisation must be aware of the pressures that your team are under on that shift at the time. Raising the issue at a meeting afterwards is too late. Document what you have done. This should include:

- the reasons for short-staffing (e.g. sickness)
- what steps you have taken to try and get further staffing (e.g. other wards, line manager, bank/agency)
- what your team have prioritised during that shift as essential and non-essential
- other actions (e.g. asked bed manager to hold admissions until next shift, etc.).

An incident form, communication book and/or e-mail to the matron/site manager will suffice as evidence that it has been documented. Keep copies.

Trying to do everything and accepting that whatever you don't get round to doing gets left is an unsafe way of working. Important care may be missed. Make a conscious decision about leaving non-essential care. Patients will not suffer if their beds are not made. If your team of staff have the time to make beds, they cannot complain that they have no time to provide adequate care.

You owe it to your staff to enable them to make these decisions in times of acute staffing shortages. Your role as a manager is to provide your staff with 'adequate and achievable demands in relation to the agreed hours of work' (Health and Safety Executive 2011). You would be failing in your duty as a manager if you were to allow your staff to continue to cope in times of acute staffing shortages without giving them the authority and skills to prioritise the aspects of care that must be left undone in order for all patients to be safe. Ensure they document and inform the appropriate senior managers of their decisions.

TAKE THE LEAD ON WARD ROUNDS

The main role for nurses taking part in ward rounds is to act as the patient's advocate by:

- ensuring the patient is involved in the discussions
- clarifying anything that the patient does not understand
- contributing to decision making on the patient's behalf
- communicating any changes or decisions to the rest of the team.

Attending ward rounds is not just about taking notes and passing the information on to the rest of the team. If that's all that were needed, you could get one of the junior doctors to hand over the list of changes afterwards, and need not attend at all.

Ensure the patient's own nurse attends the ward round

In days gone by, it was always the ward manager or nurse-in-charge that attended the ward round. Some consultants today still expect that to be the case but times have changed. Nurses no longer care for patients through the delegation of tasks from the nurse-in-charge. Nurses are now responsible for the full care of their patients, which means that they are the best people to attend the ward round.

With today's high turnover of patients and increasing patient dependency, the nurse-in-charge cannot be expected to know every detail about every patient on their ward. The role of the nurse-in-charge is therefore to ensure that the nurse who attends the ward round is the patient's own nurse, and only to take over when that nurse is unavailable.

ENSURE THE PATIENT IS INVOLVED IN DISCUSSIONS

Some health care professionals, including doctors, have a tendency to stand at the end of the bed to discuss the patient's treatment and care without including them. In any other situation, this would be considered quite rude but often the patient is too ill and too vulnerable to do anything about it. The nurse can ensure their patient is included by going to sit with them at the bedside. The rest of the ward round members would then have to turn towards the patient when liaising with the nurse. It's a simple and easy way of ensuring the patient is involved.

CLARIFY ANYTHING THAT THE PATIENT DOES NOT UNDERSTAND

When anyone starts using medical or technical terms, asking the patient if they understand is not always sufficient. Being surrounded by a group of doctors and other health care professionals can be quite overwhelming. In these circumstances, it is difficult for patients to ask the right questions. Your role is to assist their understanding, rather than just checking it. It would be far more useful for the patient if you asked them 'Would you like us to explain what the term X means?' rather than 'Do you understand?'

CONTRIBUTE TO DECISION MAKING ON THE PATIENT'S BEHALF

Your team spend more time with the patients than other health care professionals so are usually more aware of their needs than the rest of those attending the ward round. It is therefore only natural that they should contribute to all the decision making. Part of your role as ward manager should be to spend time developing the skills and confidence of your staff to enable them to speak up on behalf of the patient. Decisions should only be made with full contribution from all members of the multiprofessional team.

Observe the patients' body language

Be wary if your patient is being given too much information. They may not be able to take it all in. As their advocate, it's up to you to recognise the signs. Are they looking nervous? Arc they looking away from the person speaking to them? A simple question such as 'Are you alright?' or 'Would you prefer to discuss this part of the treatment at a later time?' should be sufficient for the patient to be able to speak up. 'Patients should be given the sense of freedom to indicate when they do not want any (or more) information: this requires skill and understanding from healthcare professionals' (Kennedy 2001; recommendation 16).

INFORMATION SHARING POST WARD ROUND

In some wards, the nurse-in-charge attends the ward round then goes round to the patients' allocated nurses and explains what decisions were made about changes in care. This is simply duplicating work and wasting precious time. It makes a lot more sense for the patient's own nurse to attend the ward round. This nurse would note any changes or decisions in the patient's care plan at the time of the ward round. The information should then be passed to everyone by having a short team brief after the ward round with all the team present.

USE WARD ROUNDS AS A LEARNING OPPORTUNITY

Whenever you can, have a junior member of staff or student to accompany you on the ward round to appreciate the art of communication. It enables them to understand that attending a ward round is far more than just taking notes. Have them observe the techniques you use in acting as the patient's advocate. Take time after the ward round to discuss what they have learned. You can send your staff on any number of communication courses, but you can't beat learning through observation and experience.

ACTION POINTS

- Ensure that you and your staff have full access to relevant and up-to-date clinical information both online and via textbooks and downloaded journal articles.
- Make sure your team are aware that full assessments and care plans are mandatory for all patients admitted to your ward.
- Include HCAs in handovers, decision-making processes and planning care if you do not already do so.
- Review your handover system if it is taking too long.
- Review the system you use for organising patient care if it does not ensure that one registered nurse is responsible for a patient's care from admission through to discharge.
- Put up information boards at the entrance to your ward to welcome all visitors, give appropriate information and invite comments/suggestions.
- Use audits, benchmarking and quality indicators to improve care but don't allow the associated paperwork to take priority over actual patient care.
- Give your staff the skills and authority to prioritise and let go of non-essential tasks in times of acute staffing shortages.
- Develop the skills of your staff in acting as the patient's advocate during ward rounds.

References

Barrett, D., Wilson, B., Woollands, A., 2009. Care planning: a guide for nurses. Pearson Education, Harlow.

Care Quality Commission, 2010. Essential standards of quality and safety. Online. Available: http://www.cqc.org.uk Feb 2012.

Healthcare Commission, 2009. Investigation into Mid Staffordshire NHS Foundation Trust. Online. Available: http://www.rcn.org.uk/__data/assets/pdf_file/0004/234976/Healthcare_Commission_report.pdf Feb 2012.

Health and Safety Executive, 2011. The management standards for work-related stress. Online. Available: http://www.hse.gov.uk/stress/standards/index.htm Feb 2012.

Kennedy, I., 2001. Learning from Bristol: the report of the public inquiry into children's heart surgery at the Bristol Royal Infirmary 1984–1995. Online. Available: http://www.bristol-inquiry.org.uk/final_report Feb 2012.

Lardner, R., 1996. Effective shift handover – a literature review. HSE, Suffolk. Online. Available: http://www.hse.gov.uk/research/otopdf/1996/oto96003.pdf Feb 2012.

NHS, 2012. The NHS brand guidelines. Online. Available: http://www.nhsidentity.nhs.uk Feb 2012.

NHS Scotland, 2011. Code of conduct for healthcare support workers. Online. Available: http://www.scotland.gov.uk/Resource/Doc/288853/0088360.pdf Feb 2012.

Nursing and Midwifery Council, 2008. The NMC code: standards for conduct, performance and ethics. NMC, London. Online. Available: http://www.nmc-uk.org Feb 2012.

Nursing and Midwifery Council, 2011. Statistics about fitness to practice hearings. Online. Available: http://www.nmc-uk.org/Hearings/Hearings-and-outcomes/Statistics-about-fitness-to-practise-hearings-/ Feb 2012.

Royal College of Nursing, 2008. Health care assistants and assistant practitioners: delegation and accountability. Online. Available: http://www.rcn.org.uk/__data/assets/pdf_file/0004/198049/HCA_booklet.pdf Feb 2012.

Thompson, D., Wright, K., 2003. Developing a unified patient record: a practical guide. Radcliffe Medical Press, Oxon.

UNISON, 2009. UNISON evidence to the pay review body: UNISON member survey. . Online. Available: http://www.unison.org.uk/acrobat/UNISON%20Evidence%20to%20NHSPRB09.pdf Feb 2012.

MANAGE YOUR BUDGET

If you manage a ward or department, then you also manage a budget. Don't let others manage it for you. You are the most appropriate person to ensure this money is used appropriately and effectively. Only you understand what the needs of the patients are on your ward, and the demands on your staff. Only you can decide on the different mix of bands and skills required within your team. And only you have an idea about the amount of equipment and consumables required.

Some ward managers say that their clinical duties are more important than the budget, but it is the budget that determines what you can and cannot do clinically. How well the budget is managed directly affects how good the care is on your ward.

KNOW WHAT YOUR BUDGET IS

It typically costs in excess of £1 million per year to run a ward. The amount obviously varies depending on the number of beds and specialty. Most ward managers claim they manage a budget but few can say what their budget is when asked. Do you know what your budget is? It is very important you are aware of how much money you are responsible for, and where and how it should be spent.

The actual figure will be shown on your monthly budget statement. It is the total amount at the bottom of the column marked 'ANNUAL BUDGET'. The budget is usually much bigger for areas such as intensive care units and accident and emergency departments.

ARE YOU MANAGING OR JUST MONITORING?

Having such a large amount of money is quite a responsibility but some make the mistake of assuming that checking through the monthly statements is all that's required. This is not managing the budget, it's simply monitoring it.

Actively managing a budget entails:

- planning how next year's budget will be spent
- keeping to specific guidelines for allocating annual leave, sickness and study leave allowances
- performing regular staffing, skill mix and workload reviews
- being fully involved in the yearly business planning process, which includes identifying cost pressures and service developments and writing business cases where necessary.

YOUR STAFFING ESTABLISHMENT

Staffing costs should be regularly revised following any changes in workload. There are several off the shelf tools currently in use for reviewing skill mix, such as GRASP (2011) and Q-Acuity (Qualitiva 2011) and the Safer Nursing Care Tool (NHS Institute for Innovation and Improvement 2009). These tools calculate the patients' care requirements in terms of staff numbers and grade mix. The measurements determine the ideal numbers and types of staff required per shift or the ideal numbers per group of beds, e.g. one nurse to five beds. A skill mix review will not automatically get you more staff, unfortunately. You need to get involved in the commissioning and business planning cycle to be able to influence your staffing levels (see p. 111).

Currently, many nurse managers use their own in-house criteria to determine their staffing numbers, such as:

- no less than two registered nurses per shift
- no less than three staff on nights
- one extra registered nurse each shift for 'theatre days', etc.

The nurse manager's intuition and common sense with regards to staffing requirements are often far better than any skill mix review.

RATIO OF NURSES TO PATIENTS

In California (USA) and Victoria (Australia), the mandatory requirement for the number of nurses to patients on medical/surgical wards is 1:5 plus one in charge

(International Council of Nurses (ICN) 2009). In the UK, there is no specific legal requirement for wards. In general, the average ratio in the UK is 1:9 patients on general wards, and 1:11 patients in wards for care of the elderly (Ball 2010). This is evidently below the practice in California or Australia – especially with research showing that the decrease in nurse:patient ratio from 1:4 to 1:8 results in a 31% increase in mortality (Aitken et al 2002) – but in spite of this, at the time of writing, there are no plans to introduce any statutory requirements in the near future.

While we do not have any statutory guidance on nursing numbers, we do have the Royal College of Nursing (RCN) guidance on the ratio of nurses to health care assistants (HCAs). This has been referred to as a 'rule of thumb' in several investigations such as that undertaken at the Mid Staffordshire NHS Trust in 2007. The RCN recommendation is that ward establishments should comprise 65% registered nurses and 35% HCAs (RCN 2006), so bear this in mind when reviewing your staffing levels with your line manager and finance advisor. Do not accept any less. Put it in writing if you are being forced to do so. The NMC code states quite clearly that 'you must report your concerns in writing if problems in the environment of care are putting people at risk' (Nursing and Midwifery Council (NMC) 2008). In England, the NHS Constitution states that patients have a right to be treated by 'appropriately qualified and experienced staff' and, in addition, demonstrating sufficient staffing is a requirement for registration with the Care Quality Commission (CQC 2010, Department of Health 2010).

MATCHING THE ROSTER TO YOUR STAFFING ESTABLISHMENT

Your staffing establishment is worked out by your finance advisor using information from your roster (i.e. the minimum staffing levels required per shift that either you have identified personally or through a formal skill-mix review). It is essential that the minimum staffing levels on your roster match the numbers in your staffing establishment. If you do not know for sure, ask your finance advisor to work it out for you.

Each directorate usually has a dedicated finance advisor. It is their job to work with you to help you ensure the budget is right for your needs. It is your job to maintain regular contact with them. If you do not, who is it they are getting their information from? And how accurate is that information?

PRIORITISE PAY

Your budget is made up of two parts:

1. PAY – this section reflects the salaries of your staff.
2. NON PAY – this section contains the money for equipment and consumables.

The PAY section takes up the first part of your budget statement. It is the part that you need to concentrate on because it usually comprises at least 80% of your total budget.

THE IMPORTANCE OF GOOD ROSTER MANAGEMENT

If your PAY budget is overspent, it can be due to inefficient rosters. To manage the PAY part of your budget effectively, you need to:

- ensure your staffing establishment matches your required 'numbers' on the roster
- manage the 20–23% allowance, which covers annual leave, study leave and unplanned absence such as sick leave
- control agency and bank usage to within the 20–23% allowance.

Staffing establishment

You will probably have set minimum staffing levels for each shift over a 7-day week (Table 6.1). The person who does the roster then allocates the staff to meet those minimum levels on each shift. Your staffing establishment (which you should receive with your monthly statement) is worked out based on your set shift requirements (Table 6.2). You must check regularly with your finance advisor that they match up. If you do not ensure that the staffing establishment meets the set shift numbers then you cannot devise the roster within budget and are therefore failing to manage it.

20–23% absence allowance (which should be built into your establishment)

When your finance advisor works out your staffing requirements, they use your roster numbers but also put in an additional 20–23% to cover annual leave, sickness/absence and study leave. It means that your final staffing establishment should

---

TABLE 6.1: Example of minimum staffing levels over 7-day week

	Mon	Tues	Wed	Thurs	Fri	Sat	Sun
Early	6	7	6	6	6	5	5
Late	6	6	6	6	5	5	5
Night	4	4	4	4	4	3	3

TABLE 6.2: Example of a ward staffing establishment

Description	Budget (WTE*)	Actual (WTE)
Ward manager (band 7)	1.0	1.0
Sister/charge nurse (band 6)	2.0	1.8
Staff nurse (band 5)	12.0	12.2
HCA (band 4)	8.0	6.0
HCA (band 3)	5.0	7.0
Ward clerk	1.0	1.0
TOTAL	29	29

*WTE, whole time equivalent; 1.00 WTE is full time, < 1.00 WTE is part time.

provide you with enough to cover your annual leave, sickness/absence and study leave requirements and remain within budget.

Sometimes some of this allowance is separated as a separate line within your budget statement and labelled as 'bank/agency costs'.

The additional 20–23% usually comprises:

- 13.5% annual leave and bank holidays (27 + 8 = 35 days)
- 1–2% study leave (2.5–5 days)
- 5–7% unplanned absences such as sickness, maternity, compassionate and carers' leave (13–18 days).

If you do not manage annual leave, sick leave and study leave correctly, you can overspend unnecessarily. Check out with your finance advisor exactly what percentage your organisation adds to cover absence allowance. Without knowing this figure, you cannot manage your PAY budget effectively.

Bank and agency usage

Use bank (NHS Professionals in England) instead of agency wherever possible. They cost little more than permanent staff. If you are sent an agency nurse because no bank nurses are available, an additional 33% is usually charged in commission to the agency. This means that for every three shifts covered by agency staff, one shift should remain unfilled in order to make up for the extra cost. Obviously this needs to be handled very carefully because, at the same time, you cannot compromise patient care. Some managers compensate for the extra commission charges by booking agency nurses for a 'half shift' only.

In some organisations, the most popular shifts for bank staff are early shifts. This means that the late and night shifts are covered by agency. It therefore makes sense to compile rosters to ensure that most late and night shifts are covered by your own staff, leaving the vacant shifts mainly as early shifts. This will ensure that there is a higher chance of getting bank staff rather than agency.

'BUDDY UP' WITH ANOTHER WARD

Try and work closely with another ward manager and share staff between your two wards during the hard times. It is advisable to link up with another ward or department with a similar specialty within your directorate for the purpose of sharing staff. You could meet with the manager once per week to go through the next week's roster. This enables you to identify areas where resources could be shared and to plan ahead for expected shortfalls.

BE FLEXIBLE WITH YOUR STAFFING ESTABLISHMENT

Be more flexible with your staffing establishment. If you are unable to recruit a certain grade of staff into your vacant post, then consider other options. Can you replace with a different grade of staff? Think carefully; perhaps it would be better to employ an available lower grade of staff rather than fill the vacancy continually with bank and agency.

As the budget holder, you do not have to stick to the grades of staff in your budget statement. You can adjust them according to the needs of the ward and what's available so long as you remain within budget. Your finance advisor's role is to assist you in doing so and they will calculate any differences for you. You will also need your line manager's overall approval.

GO THROUGH YOUR MONTHLY BUDGET STATEMENT

The budget statement tells what you have spent. It's like going through your own bank statement at the end of the month. Nothing should come as a surprise. It should confirm what you already know.

The layout of the budget statement varies between organisations. However, the information contained is basically the same. It is usually divided into two parts, PAY and NON PAY, and is best read using the following columns.

Establishment (budget)

This column tells you how many staff you can employ within your budget (WTE stands for 'whole time equivalent': 1.0 WTE is full time, and anything less than 1.0 WTE is part time (e.g. 0.6 WTE equates to funding for someone to work 3 days per week).

Establishment (actual)

This column tells you how many staff you have in post. The numbers will vary. For example, if you cannot recruit up to establishment in band 6, you can recruit more in band 5 to compensate, as long as the final salary figure remains the same.

Code

This is the finance code given to each particular grade of staff or type of equipment. The first part of the code relates to your ward (usually a 4-digit number). The second part relates to the category of staff or equipment (usually another 4-digit number).

Annual budget

This is usually the last column on the right hand side of your budget statement. The numbers in this column never change. It tells you what money you have to spend over the whole year. You should be very familiar with these figures.

Current month's budget, expenditure and variance

These three columns tell you what you had to spend in the last month (budget), what you did spend (expenditure) and what the difference is (variance).

Year to date's budget, expenditure and variance

These three columns tell you what you have had in your budget so far since the beginning of the financial year (budget), what you have spent in that time (expenditure) and where you are at the moment in terms of overall under-spend or over-spend (variance).

CHECKING THROUGH THE COLUMNS

When you receive your budget statement, the first thing you need to do is check the total amount in the 'year to date' variance column. It tells you how over-spent or under-spent you are at the moment. Remember to concentrate on the PAY section, as this is usually the part where most of your budget is allocated.

If you have an over-spend, take a look at the rest of this column to find out which bit is over-spent. Over-spends should not be a surprise. You know when you have used extra agency to cover high sickness levels or have had an unexpected increase in workload in the past month. The key to managing your budget effectively is deciding what to do about this over-spend. You should have already warned your line manager and finance manager, and together worked out a plan of action to bring the budget back in line. If not, it is advisable to do so at this point.

You also need to check the first two columns in the PAY section (i.e. budgeted and actual establishment) for accuracy. It is often the case that a 'leavers' form may not have been processed when a member of staff leaves or transfers to another ward. If this happens, your ward will continue to fund their pay until the form is processed.

Overall, your main task with the budget statement is to check for any inaccuracies and identify the main variances. You should then discuss your findings with your financial advisor each month and write a plan of action for the coming month.

INVOLVE YOUR TEAM

Go through your budget statement with your staff regularly. Get feedback from those who have responsibility for aspects of the NON PAY (see p. 110). Discuss and agree actions for both PAY and NON PAY. Sharing the budget statements with your team helps in their development and ensures they appreciate the links between good budgeting and good patient care.

MANAGE ANNUAL LEAVE

CALCULATING THE ANNUAL LEAVE ALLOWANCE PER ROSTER

The average percentage given for annual leave is usually 13.5%. This equates to 35 days (27 + 8) per person. In order to manage this annual leave allowance effectively, you have to make sure that a certain number of staff are on annual leave at any one time. Generally, 13.5% of your establishment equates to around one in every seven staff. In other words, for every seven staff in your team, one should be on annual leave. This ensures that annual leave is spread throughout the year so that adequate numbers of staff are available to work at all times.

SPREADING ANNUAL LEAVE THROUGHOUT THE YEAR

Poor staffing levels between January and March due to high levels of annual leave indicate that the ward manager has not managed their budget properly. They will be over-spent as a consequence. Encourage your staff to take annual leave regularly throughout the year and book this at least 4 weeks in advance of the roster. The following guidelines are generally recommended (check with your local organisational guidelines):

- By end-June – minimum of 1 week must have been taken.
- By end-Sept – minimum of 3 weeks must have been taken.
- By end-Dec – minimum of 5 weeks must have been taken.
- Jan to end-Mar – maximum of 1 week of annual leave to be taken.

A good tip is to keep an annual leave planner on the wall in the ward office with separate annual leave lines for the number of staff who can take annual leave at any one time. Staff can then fill in the slots where they want to take annual leave over the coming year. You can also see at a glance what is happening and be able to intervene if necessary. It will stop staff leaving it to the last minute to book and finding out there are no annual leave slots left.

If any of your staff wish to carry annual leave allowance over into the next financial year, you should clarify first how you can allow for this within the following year's budget.

Try not to resort to allocating annual leave. It is better to take time to explain to your team how the budget and annual leave allowance are so closely linked. Get them to understand that if they don't book their annual leave early and spread it out over the year, it will cause an over-spend in the budget and you will end up having to make other cutbacks (e.g. stopping bank and agency) to bring it back in line.

MANAGE YOUR UNPLANNED ABSENCE ALLOWANCE

You usually have an allowance of up to 7% for unplanned absence such as sick leave, maternity leave, carers' leave, etc. (check what your own organisation allows): 7% equates to around 18 days of unplanned absence per person per year without incurring an over-spend. This does not mean that each person can take 18 days off sick per year! It means that you have enough funding to cover an overall absence rate (due to sickness, maternity, carers' or compassionate leave) in your team of up to 7% without going over budget.

Make sure you have systems in place to monitor sickness rates closely. You need to be able to look at trends over time. It is not enough to get a 'feel' for the level of absence. Calculate it at the end of each completed roster. In some organisations, particularly those using e-rostering, the ward managers are sent a summary of their staff sickness rates each month. If your organisation does not have this system in place, you can easily work it out for yourself using the equation outlined in Box 6.1.

BOX 6.1: CALCULATING STAFF SICKNESS RATES

Number of days lost ÷ number of days rostered × 100 = sickness percentage.
Example: If Nurse Smith was rostered to work 20 days during the last roster but was off sick for four of them:

$$4 \div 20 \times 100 = 20\%$$

The time lost by Nurse Smith was 20% of her potential working time.

TABLE 6.3: Example of record of staff sickness on ward at 6 months

Staff	Shifts rostered	Shifts off sick	% Sickness	Episodes
Rose	120	6	5 %	3
Emma	122	8	6.5 %	2
Jane	120	2	1.7 %	1
Susan	119	0	0 %	0
Amy	120	5	4.2 %	1
Gemma	121	0	0 %	0
Dave	120	2	1.7 %	1
John	100	0	0 %	0
TOTAL	942	23	2.4 %	8

Total no. of shifts lost to sickness ÷ Total no. of shifts rostered = $23 \div 942 \times 100$
Total percentage of sickness to date = 2.4%

On completion of each 4-week roster, it is advisable to keep and update a continuous record of the team's sickness rates (Table 6.3).

SICKNESS MONITORING

You should be able to demonstrate that you are taking action where sickness levels are high. If the sickness rates go beyond your organisation's target level, you need to look at the reasons and take action to reduce them. If the main reason for sickness is due to back problems, for example, then it would be wise to undertake further moving and handling risk assessments, involve the manual handling advisor and invest extra funding into moving and handling training/equipment.

MATERNITY LEAVE

The percentage for unplanned absence usually incorporates maternity leave. If the maternity leave is particularly high within your department, you need to highlight this with your general manager who will have the authority to transfer funding between departments if necessary.

Some organisations hold the maternity leave budget centrally. If this is the case, you must ensure the allowance is allocated to your budget when affected by maternity leave. This can be achieved through close liaison and monitoring with your line manager and finance advisor.

OTHER LEAVE

With the increasing emphasis on family-friendly and flexible working policies, there are now other types of leave that you need to manage carefully within your allowance for unplanned absences. These include paternity leave, time off to attend antenatal classes, adoption leave, carers' leave and compassionate leave. Keep a running check on how much all this leave is costing you. You may have to apply for more to be added in your budget.

PLAN YOUR STUDY LEAVE ALLOWANCE

You usually have an allowance within the budget of around 1–2% for covering study leave (some organisations allocate more, some less, so you must check exactly what you have with your finance advisor). This equates to between 2 and 5 days per staff member per year. This does not mean that each member of your team is entitled to be released for this number of study days per year. The study leave allowance should be viewed as a total for the whole team of staff. For example, if you have a team of 30 WTE, 2% study leave allowance would give you up to 150 study days per year that can be granted to your team ($30 \times 5 = 150$ days).

The study leave allowance needs to be planned carefully at around November time in the preceding financial year, taking the following steps:

1. Multiply the total number of your budgeted WTE establishment by the number of study days your organisation allocates per WTE, which will give the total number of days that can be allocated for study leave over the coming financial year (as outlined in the example above).
2. Identify all the study needs of all staff in your team (via the annual appraisal process) in terms of mandatory requirements plus professional and personal development needs
3. Find out exactly what the study leave requirements are for each course that staff members have identified.
4. Total the amount of study leave that your staff will require for the coming year.
5. If the total study leave required is more than the total number of shifts allowed in your budget, priorities have to be made. A good way to decide these priorities is to ask your team. Use a team meeting to get them to decide among themselves who gets priority. Facilitate the discussion to ensure it is done in a fair and consistent manner.

It is always advisable to keep a portion of the study leave allowance aside to be used for unexpected courses, workshops or seminars that may arise throughout the year, which would benefit the staff and service. If extra courses come up during the year that do not come within the 1–2% allowance, replacement costs must be identified from another source, unless the workload means you can 'go down' on numbers, or the member of staff concerned is willing to go in their own (unpaid) time.

OTHER SOURCES OF FUNDING

Keep close links with the manager of your organisation's training and development department and with your link university. This will help keep you aware of any further 'pots' of money that become available throughout the year (often at the end of each financial year between January and March). Various charities such as the

League of Friends will sometimes support staff for training courses. You have to find out where these extra funds are; they tend not to be generally advertised.

MANDATORY TRAINING

Include all mandatory training within your allowance. If you are not careful, mandatory training days can use up all your study leave allowance. The staff in the training department may not realise this. It is up to you and your colleagues to point it out to them and present an alternative solution. Some organisations have condensed their training into short 2-hour sessions, which can either be put together to cover three to four subjects in one day or held as separate sessions during the afternoon handover period.

Study leave needs to be carefully controlled. Keeping your staff informed and fully involved in the process of allocation helps them to understand the restrictions you are working to and reduces any feelings of resentment about study leave allocation.

GET YOUR STAFF INVOLVED IN NON PAY

The NON PAY part of your budget is usually set out in the second part of your budget statement. The only difference between PAY and NON PAY on the statement is that the establishment and WTE columns will remain blank because NON PAY does not involve people. The overall amount you have in NON PAY is usually far less than the PAY section. The list of items may be longer but this does not mean it is more important. It is just easier to ascertain where the money has gone.

NON PAY may appear to be your lower priority but it still needs tight control. A good way to manage it is to delegate each budget line to a member of your staff. This will give them a good insight into budget management and helps them to develop budgeting skills with appropriate support. The main ones to delegate are pharmacy/drugs, medical supplies and stationery. These usually have another separate list showing more minute details of the expenditure that your staff can manage, leaving you to concentrate on the PAY budget, which is your biggest expenditure.

PHARMACY/DRUGS

The nurse responsible for this budget would probably form close links with the ward pharmacist. Their role would include going through the monthly pharmacy budget in detail and becoming familiar with what is being used, what is needed and any changes that are being made. They would be able to identify any cost pressures (see p. 111), such as new routine drugs introduced during the current financial year, that were not originally budgeted for.

MEDICAL SUPPLIES

Most hospitals nowadays rely on a top-up system. Allocating one member of your team to monitor usage and trends will help keep the stock levels appropriate to what is needed and identify any unnecessary expenditure. They will also be able to liaise with the appropriate company representatives (alongside NHS supplies if working within the NHS) to keep abreast of what's new and perhaps more appropriate for your group of patients.

STATIONERY

The stationery budget is often best delegated to your ward receptionist who is usually the most appropriate person to know what is being used and where to make savings.

BE MORE ACTIVE IN THE BUSINESS PLANNING PROCESS

Get involved with the business planning process for your directorate. The budgets are reset each year as part of the annual business planning process cycle (which in turn takes account of predicted levels of activity and decisions made by the commissioning groups). It's something with which you should be familiar as the budget holder. Some ward managers are left out of this important process. It's up to you to make sure you get involved. Ward budgets can be inappropriate if someone else is deciding what your ward needs.

The process usually begins around November every year in the NHS when all wards and departments in your organisation have to identify what they need for the next year. The whole process takes up to 6 months (remember, each financial year is from April 1st to March 31st). The general manager's role is to produce the final business plan which represents all the wards and departments in their directorate. The final plan outlines to the board what funding is required to manage the service in the coming year. It includes any extra funding required due to changes in the service.

The director of finance together with the other board directors agree how much each directorate will get based on the business plans which the general managers have submitted and the levels of activity and decisions made by the trust's commissioners. It's the general manager's role to write the full business plan, not yours. You are a nurse manager, not a business manager. However, you do need to contribute to the process.

THE BUSINESS PLAN

Your general manager is usually tasked with identifying the *cost pressures* and *service developments* through all their department leads:

● A *cost pressure* is an approved change that has already happened over the past year, which needs funding for the future to *maintain existing service levels*, e.g. equipment that requires updating/replacing or a nationally approved pay rise for staff.

- A *service development* is an authorised planned change that will be needed to *improve the quantity or quality of service* in the future, e.g. the implementation of a patient follow-up service or the appointment of a nurse specialist.

The general manager usually has to produce evidence for each item in the form of a business case. This is the stage where you need to ensure you are not left out. If you need another member of staff due to increased turnover of patients, then you have to present a 'business case'. Do this together with your line manager and finance advisor, who will work out all the costs for you.

If you do not do this, either:

- someone else will do it for you; this might be someone who may not understand the service as well as you and therefore will not present your case so well, or
- your needs will not be added to the overall business plan.

There are usually too many cost pressures and service developments so priorities have to be made. Some will be rejected because there is simply not enough money for them all. If you are not involved and don't get across to your general manager the importance of your needs then you will probably not get them.

HOW TO WRITE A BUSINESS CASE

There is no point in writing a business case if:

- your manager does not agree and has no intention of agreeing to include it in the overall business plan, or
- your manager feels that the funding could be sought elsewhere.

A business case is simply a way of presenting evidence that the item is really needed. Many organisations provide a business case form to be completed in each case. Box 6.2 gives an example of the information that is generally required.

DON'T DO ANYTHING WITHOUT IDENTIFIED FUNDING

It is imperative that you do not implement anything new at all without the identified funding. As mentioned previously, nurses have a wonderful ability to cope when under-resourced. Unfortunately this leads to more problems than it solves. If you can take on extra work without extra resources, then why would the organisation give you further funding?

If you are already providing an extra service without extra funding, you have to take action to ensure the funding is put into the following year's budget. (For example, if you have a couple of HCAs who have automatically been given a pay increase for achieving NVQ level 3, but no budget had been set aside for this, it would be classified as a cost pressure.) In the meantime, look at what service you will cease to provide in order to provide the extra service within budget. (For example, you can alter the staffing establishment to meet the extra cost of the HCAs' increased salary.)

BOX 6.2: EXAMPLE OF A FORMAT FOR WRITING A BUSINESS CASE

Title

Explain as fully as you can within the title. Include the cost here (e.g. replacement ECG machine @ £5000 or 1 × band 5 nurse @ £30 000).

Introduction

Give a brief summary of what the problem is, the solution, why and what is the cost. Ensure you state clearly how much this initial outlay will save you in the long term.

Background

Explain the background but remember that non-clinical people may be reviewing this so you should assume that they know nothing about it. Explain what the benefits will be and what will happen if you do not get it. Your case will be much stronger if you can relate it to government targets, policy or standards (e.g. CQC, Commissioning for Quality and Innovation (CQUIN)). Also include risk assessment results where possible. In England, all business plans should link with the Operating Framework, which is a set of national priorities issued by the Department of Health each year.

Options analysis

First, describe your current service and then list all the options that could be taken, and for each of them give a brief outline including advantages, risk, constraints, potential impact, outcomes and decision (i.e. accept/reject with reasons). If possible, include a cost–benefit analysis (e.g. what would the more expensive one provide as opposed to the cheaper version?). Include the option of no change. What would happen if you do nothing? Try to talk in numbers as much as possible (e.g. how much it would cost in terms of nursing hours spent going round other wards each day to borrow an ECG machine). Your finance advisor will work out the costings for you. How many patients would suffer? How many may have treatment delayed? What care standard will you not meet?

Preferred option

State your preferred option and say why. Also list all the items that make up your final cost figure. Don't forget to include time and people. Include any savings that will be made (e.g. reduced cost of calling out facilities to fix the ECG machine every few weeks, reduced re-admission rates with an extra member of staff). It's your finance advisor's role to work out the costs for you.

Recommendations

Conclude with your recommendation(s).

Always involve your finance advisor. Being refused a cost pressure does not give you the automatic right to over-spend because you have the service anyway. You have to make savings elsewhere within your budget.

GET IT IN WRITING

Don't take on extra work with verbal promises of extra funding. Ensure you have some sort of written confirmation. It's not uncommon for ward managers to open extra beds or be persuaded to provide staff cover for clinics on the promise that funding will follow, only to find that the funding never materialises. The new service soon becomes established and cannot be withdrawn or patient care will suffer. Don't let yourself get into such a situation. Becoming wise to the business planning process reduces the risk of being duped into taking on work without appropriate funding.

If it does happen (e.g. your line manager may have agreed on your behalf to a change without realising the extra work involved and it is too late for the decision to be reversed), moaning and whingeing will not help. You should take action quickly by identifying which aspects of your existing workload must be cut in order to provide the new service. Let your manager know your decision in writing (e-mail is sufficient). Don't try to cope and allow your staff to become exhausted and stressed by trying to provide extra services without the appropriate resources. To do so amounts to poor management.

MEET REGULARLY WITH YOUR FINANCE ADVISOR

It is essential that you meet with your financial advisor regularly to:

1. *Ensure that any inaccuracies in your budget are rectified.* If you have been charged for something that you have not used, it is your financial advisor's job to get the money transferred back to your budget, but you have to identify it first. Unprocessed 'starters' and 'leavers' forms are a common source of inaccuracies that need to be identified and corrected quickly.
2. *Ensure that your staffing establishment always matches the limits set on your roster.* This is essential for good budget management. Each time a member of your staff resigns, review the job with your team (see p. 143). Don't always replace 'like with like' as the workload or skill requirement may have changed. Your finance advisor will be able to advise how you could achieve the change within your current staffing establishment but still remain within budget.
3. *Check that you are using bank and agency wisely.* If you are using them just to cover staff vacancies, there should be no over-spend. If you are using bank and agency to cover sickness, there should not be an over-spend unless your sickness levels are above the sickness allowance that was added to your budget.
4. *Calculate and prepare for any predicted over-spends.* Obviously there will be unforeseen costs such as an outbreak of MRSA or a patient who requires one-to-one care for some time. These types of extra costs are not included within your budget but you do need to monitor them closely. Simply saying 'we are over-spent because it's been busy' is insufficient. It will appear that you are not managing your budget properly. It's far better to report that 'we have a predicted overspend of £6000 this month due to the extra staffing required to special a high-dependency patient for 7 days because there were no available beds in HDU'. You must see your finance advisor early so they can forecast the extra cost to your budget. You can then work together with them and your line manager to plan how you can get your budget back on line over the rest of the financial year.
5. *Help you prepare a business case should you require more staff or equipment.* Remember that you will need your general manager's agreement before you go ahead and compile a business case.

It is the finance manager's role to provide specialist expertise and support you in managing the budget. But they will not come to you. Be proactive. Go to them and seek their advice. They are not clinically trained and often do not understand the complexities of running a ward. You are not a finance expert and do not understand the intricacies of how hospital finance works. Work together and use each other's skills to ensure your budget is managed efficiently and effectively, thus ensuring a high standard of patient care.

ACTION POINTS

- Meet with your finance advisor to confirm that your roster numbers match the staffing establishment, ensure you know the percentage of absence allowance and go through your budget statement explaining anything that you do not understand.
- Follow up with regular appointments throughout the year, preferably monthly. Go through your budget statement and discuss any problems and any changes you wish to make.
- Calculate how many staff should be on annual leave each week, and ensure all future rosters are compiled with the right numbers of staff on annual leave.
- Starting from this year, plan your next year's study leave quota in advance with your team.
- If your HR team does not supply you with monthly sickness figures for your team, maintain your own records for now.
- Delegate some NON PAY budget lines to your staff for professional development purposes, and to allow you to concentrate on PAY.
- Have a look at last year's business plan and ask your general manager to go through it with you, explaining anything you do not understand. Get involved with next year's plan and put forward your team's needs.
- Review the budget in all your team meetings. Explain and involve the team in issues such as annual leave and study leave allowances.
- Involve your staff in all decisions such as who gets study leave and where to make cost savings.
- Don't take on extra work without written confirmation of funding.

References

Aitken, L., Clarke, S., Sloane, D., et al., 2002. Hospital nurse staffing and patient mortality, nurse burnout and job satisfaction. JAMA 288, 1987–1993.

Ball, J., 2010. Guidance on safe nurse staffing levels in the UK. RCN, London. Online. Available: http://www.rcn.org.uk/__data/assets/pdf_file/0005/353237/003860.pdf Feb 2012.

Care Quality Commission, 2010. Essential standards of quality and safety. Guidance about compliance. Online. Available: http://www.cqc.org.uk/guidanceforprofessionals/nhstrusts/complyingwiththeregulations/guidanceaboutcompliance.cfm Feb 2012.

Department of Health, 2010. The NHS Constitution. Online. Available: http://www.dh.gov.uk/en/Publicationsandstatistics/Publications/PublicationsPolicyAndGuidance/DH_113613 Feb 2012.

GRASP, 2011. Skill mix analysis. Online. Available: http://www.graspinc.com/Services/SkillMix.aspx Feb 2012.

International Council of Nurses, 2009. Nursing matters factsheet: nurse:patient ratios. ICN, Geneva. Online. Available: http://www.icn.ch/images/stories/documents/publications/fact_sheets/9c_FS-Nurse_Patient_Ratio.pdf Feb 2012.

NHS Institute for Innovation and Improvement, 2009. The Safer Nursing Care tool. Online. Available: http://www.institute.nhs.uk/quality_and_value/introduction/safer_nursing_care_tool.html Feb 2012.

Nursing and Midwifery Council, 2008. The NMC code: standards for conduct, performance and ethics. NMC, London. Online. Available: http://www.nmc-uk.org Feb 2012.

Qualitiva, 2011. Q-Acuity Nursing Acuity Data Tool. Online. Available: http://www.qualitiva.com/Product-Solutions-Healthcare-Q-Acuity.aspx Feb 2012.

Royal College of Nursing, 2006. Policy guidance 15/2006: setting appropriate ward nurse staffing in NHS acute trusts. RCN, London. Online. Available: http://www.rcn.org.uk/__data/assets/pdf_file/0007/287710/setting_appropriate_ward_nurse_staffing_levels_in_nhs_acut.pdf Feb 2012.

IMPROVE QUALITY AND SAFETY

Clinical governance is an umbrella term given to all the systems that need to be in place to improve clinical quality. Currently there are many systems in the NHS which ensure that we measure and improve quality. One could argue the NHS is being audited to death at the moment, but it is necessary in the current financial climate to ensure that we are being as efficient and as effective as we can within available resources. However, you are responsible for a team of nurses, not a team of auditors. Do take care to ensure that the *measurement* of quality does not interfere with the *delivery* of quality patient care.

Quality indicators are not the only way of measuring quality. Patient surveys, comments, complaints and incidents also give us a good deal of information about where to target resources to improve our service. This chapter explains the process of quality monitoring and improvement as well as the practical tasks of dealing with complaints and incidents.

QUALITY INDICATORS

In the current climate, it seems that we are being overrun with quality indicators, which have a tendency to increase quality in one area but with the unfortunate side effect of reducing quality in another, leading to the identification of another quality indicator that has to be met and so on. An example of this is the 4-hour waiting target in A&E, which led to increased pressure on beds and the subsequent mixing of male and female patients which in turn led to problems with privacy and dignity. This in turn, has led to a number of further quality indicators for single sex wards and various other initiatives for increasing privacy and dignity. Another example is the changing of ward layouts to single rooms and 4–6-bed bays to meet hygiene, privacy and dignity indicators, resulting in the reduced ability of nurses to adequately observe and supervise and thereby contributing to an increased number of falls. Quality indicators have therefore been introduced to reduce the number of falls, including initiatives such as hourly rounding. And so it goes on …

Sometimes, we can be so taken with the need to meet quality indicators that we allow them to override our common sense and clinical priorities. Remember that, first and foremost, you are a clinician and the patients' needs are your priority. This is particularly pertinent at times when you have to choose between meeting a quality indicator and ensuring that patients get appropriate individualised care. An example would be the choice between getting a patient discharged by 12 noon or taking the time to ensure they understand their discharge medication. To be able to make an appropriate choice, you should have some idea of what the most important quality indicators are, where they come from and why they are so important.

CARE QUALITY COMMISSION (CQC)

In England, all health care providers – both NHS and private – have to be registered with the CQC, which has a number of quality indicators that have to be met, called the Essential Standards of Quality and Safety (CQC 2010). If any part of your organisation does not meet these standards, the CQC has the power to temporarily suspend work or even shut down that department. At the time of writing, the CQC has already shut down 34 care homes and 8 agencies that did not meet the standards. They do, of course, give organisations adequate notice to improve first.

The systems in Scotland, Wales and Northern Ireland all vary slightly from this. For example, the Scottish Healthcare Inspectorate focuses on quality indicators for reducing infection rates and inspects each local health board twice every 3 years. NHS Wales improves quality through the 1000 Lives Plus programme and through locally agreed targets.

Many of the quality indicators used are heavily influenced by the National Institute for Health and Clinical Excellence (NICE) guidance in England and Wales. Scotland and Northern Ireland differ in that they usually (but not always) disseminate the NICE guidance but only after reviewing it first.

COMMISSIONING FOR QUALITY AND INNOVATION (CQUIN)

In addition to the CQC performance indicators in England, the commissioning groups also set certain quality indicators that have to be met. When they commission (i.e. agree to buy for a certain price) services from hospitals, they attach some quality indicators, and if these are not met, they can withhold a percentage of the total payment. Quality indicators used so far include areas such as the percentage of patients who have had a venous thromboembolism (VTE) risk assessment on admission, the percentage of 12-noon discharges and the percentage of surgical site infections.

One good way of influencing such decisions is to find a way of becoming involved in the commissioning process. For example, some commissioning groups are stating what the staff to patient ratio requirements should be for their patients when admitted to certain units. There are various databases of quality indicators from which the commissioning groups can pick and choose. These include 'nurse-sensitive outcome indicators', which were previously known as 'nursing metrics' (NHS Information Centre 2011). They can also choose to include the indicators produced by the various initiatives outlined in the following section. At the time of writing, NHS Scotland are currently developing a specific database of clinical quality indicators (CQIs) for nursing.

NURSING QUALITY INDICATORS

There are various other quality initiatives in nursing, which include the following:

- *Quality, Innovation, Productivity and Prevention (QIPP)* – A set of 12 'workstreams' (subjects) such as end-of-life care and long-term conditions, chosen because of the need to improve efficiency and effectiveness.
- *The Productive Series* – A set of initiatives for eliminating waste and reducing costs based on the successful use of similar initiatives in the car manufacturing industry.
- *High Impact Actions* – A set of specific areas for concentrating action to improve quality, such as improving nutrition levels, and preventing falls, pressure ulcers, infections and delayed discharges.
- *Essence of Care* – A set of benchmarks for wards and departments to use to share and compare practice, ensuring that they all meet the same high standard.

The above list is just a small sample of the plethora of quality initiatives being implemented across England at the time of writing this book. In 2010, they were all incorporated under one framework called 'Energise for Excellence' (E4E) (see Box 7.1). Many are simply ways of trying to save money but without *reducing* quality. QIPP, for example, was specifically tailored to meet the £20 billion savings required by the government to be made by 2015.

It is important to 'keep an eye' as to what is going on and where the various quality indicators come from. You also need to be fully aware of the penalty that comes with the non-completion of each quality indicator. There may be times when you have to choose one quality indicator over another in terms of reaching the standard, particularly when staffing shortages become acute.

BOX 7.1: ENERGISE FOR EXCELLENCE IN CARE

1. Get staffing right.
2. Deliver quality nursing and midwifery care.
3. Measure the impact of nursing and midwifery care.
4. Improved patient experience.
5. Improved staff experience.

(Department of Health 2010)

IDENTIFY MISTAKES AND RISKS

There will always be an element of risk within health care because things are always changing and no change comes without risk. Managing risk is therefore a continuous process. Standards, policies and procedures are continually being updated to reduce the risk of things going wrong but inevitably no system or human being is perfect and mistakes will continue to be made. We currently have a National Reporting and Learning System (NRLS) originally set up by the National Patient Safety Agency (NPSA) in 2003, which gathers data from all health care organisations in England and Wales (Northern Ireland and Scotland operate more local systems of reporting and data collection). The NRLS distributes the learning from these data via patient safety alerts, guidelines and policies. We also have a system of dealing with complaints that ensures they are investigated locally, recurring themes are identified and improvements made accordingly.

As the ward manager, you should be familiar with the systems for dealing with complaints and incidents. This will ensure that you do not get weighed down with bureaucracy, are able to support your staff and the patients and relatives involved, and focus on making improvements to care as a direct result.

BE OPEN AND SAY SORRY

Generally, all patients want is an apology, an explanation of what went wrong and reassurance that mistakes will not recur, yet nearly half of all the complaints upheld by the Health Service Ombudsman in 2010 were because an apology was not given. 'When things do go wrong, an apology can be a powerful remedy; simple to deliver and costing nothing' (Parliamentary and Health Service Ombudsman 2010).

Saying sorry is not an admission of liability (NHS Litigation Authority (NHSLA) 2009); in fact, there have been various studies from hospitals in Australia, Singapore and the USA that have shown a marked reduction in the number of claims since policies were introduced that promote the concept of saying sorry when things go wrong (NPSA 2009). Do ensure that your team are all aware of this. Most organisations now have guidelines for staff on how to communicate with patients and their families when a mistake has been made, particularly when any harm has been caused. One recommendation for ensuring a good apology is to refer to the three Rs recommended by Armstrong (2010):

- Regret – say sorry.
- Reason – be honest and explain that it was unintentional.
- Remedy – explain the next steps such as investigation and feedback.

SUPPORT YOUR STAFF

Working in health care is a vocation and we are all dedicated professionals. To give care to others every day sometimes under very difficult circumstances and then be the subject of a complaint or an incident investigation can be soul-destroying. It needs to be handled very sensitively. All health care professionals are naturally going to feel upset and perhaps even angry. They may feel that they have given so much yet all they get in return is a written complaint or a demand for a statement about areas of care that may have been missed. Try to remember that these are not formal disciplinary or performance management procedures. They are informal and designed to help us learn and improve our services. Formal, signed witness statements are not required for either complaint or incident investigations.

If a particular individual is involved, then it would be better for you to investigate and handle the complaint or incident personally rather than delegating to another member of staff. Individuals who are the subject of a complaint or incident investigation need to feel that they are fully supported by their manager. You must ensure that you:

- don't take sides during an investigation, either with the patient or the health care professional
- reassure the individual that you are not interested in blaming anyone and you just want to find out if there is anything that can be done to improve the situation
- do not hesitate to ask for advice if the situation is a particularly difficult one.

At all times, ensure that such individuals are kept involved and informed. They should see the final complaint response letter or incident report before it is sent back to the appropriate manager. It would be unfair not to let them see this and to have the chance to correct any inaccuracies. Do also reassure all staff that they will not be personally identified in any incident report.

Don't feel that you have to handle a difficult complaint or incident by yourself. The complaints manager is usually very experienced in most types of complaint and will be able to advise. The risk manager will also be able to help with any incident investigation. If you feel you need more professional support then contact your director of nursing who, in many organisations, also has executive responsibility for clinical governance and quality. They usually have a lot of experience in handling complex complaints and incidents.

KNOW WHEN TO STOP AN INCIDENT OR COMPLAINT INVESTIGATION

Discovery of significant issues/serious failures

All complaints are risk-assessed on arrival at your complaints department. If the risk is assessed as highly serious, it should be referred to a more senior manager and a root cause analysis investigation will have to be undertaken. This means that your role would probably be as part of the investigation team and someone else will have responsibility for the overall complaint response. The complaints that you receive should be those that have been assessed as low or medium in terms of seriousness. The same goes for incident investigations. They will all be graded and any serious incidents requiring investigation (SIRIs) will be handed over to a more senior manager for investigation.

However, if you discover during the course of your investigation that there are significant issues regarding standards, safeguarding or denial of rights, or serious issues such as grossly substandard care causing serious harm, you must refer it to your line manager for consideration of a separate investigation process.

When disciplinary action may be necessary

As previously mentioned, the complaints and incident procedures are entirely different from performance management and disciplinary procedures and must always be kept separate. You must stop the complaint or incident investigation process if you suspect any of the following:

- professional misconduct
- negligence
- criminal activity.

If you feel disciplinary action may be required then you must alert your line manager. A formal investigation into the matter can then be arranged.

The patient or relative involved in the complaint or incident will be informed about what is happening and that you will not be continuing with the process until you have the outcome of the alternative investigation. Never do this on your own. It requires the authority of someone more senior within your organisation. If the individual's involvement only forms one aspect of a complaint or incident, you should be able to continue to investigate the other aspects, but you cannot do both investigations at the same time. Incident and complaint investigations are informal in that they are not punitive. The disciplinary process is very formal.

INVESTIGATE COMPLAINTS APPROPRIATELY

The main aim of the NHS complaints procedures across the UK is to achieve 'local resolution'. This means that complainants should have their verbal or written complaint dealt with locally by the organisation which was treating them. If not satisfied with the written response, the complainant can take it to a second, more formal, stage. There are different procedures for the second stage depending on where in the UK the problem arose. It usually involves either asking for an 'independent review' or going straight to the Health Service Ombudsman.

This section focuses only on 'local resolution' because it is this part of the complaints process which involves the ward manager. It consists of either a verbal response to a verbal complaint, or a written response to a verbal or written complaint. It may also consist of a meeting with the complainant followed by a letter.

VERBAL COMPLAINTS

Wherever possible, verbal complaints should be dealt with immediately. A record of the conversation should include:

- the date and time
- who was present
- what information was given
- any apologies made
- any action that was taken at the time or future action you promised to undertake.

If the complaint was resolved at the time or within 1 working day, it can be regarded as resolved and closed. It's a good idea to send a copy of your notes to the complaints manager. Many hospital policies now state that *all* comments, concerns and complaints should be formally noted and a record sent to the complaints department, but be realistic: a 2-hour visiting period on a shift with staffing shortages could result in many hours of paperwork if you took that too literally! However, it should definitely be done if it is suspected that the complainant may wish to consider taking the matter further, or if it has been specifically requested.

If the verbal complaint is not resolved within 1 day, then it should be dealt with using the same procedure as that of a written complaint. All written complaints must go through the complaints department.

WRITTEN COMPLAINTS

All written complaints should be addressed to the chief executive or complaints manager. If you receive one directly you must forward it immediately to the complaints department. They will send an acknowledgement to the complainant and sort out various aspects such as permission to access the patient's notes for investigation. Once you have received a written complaint from the complaints department with a request to respond, the following four steps are recommended:

1. Check you understand exactly what the complaint is about and what the complainant expects from you. In many organisations, a member of staff in the complaints department will have called the complainant and done this for you already. They will agree a plan with the complainant and forward it on to you. However, if you are not clear from the plan what they mean, call the complaints department to clarify or contact the complainant. Maintaining personal contact

in the early stages will help ensure the complainant is confident that something is being done. It is positively encouraged through national policy to keep in contact with the complainant throughout the process.

2. Appoint and support a member of your team to help you investigate (your staff need the experience).
3. Once you have sufficient information, write a response/report or organise a meeting with the complainant and follow up with a letter.
4. Discuss the complaint, and any learning/actions from the investigation process, with your team.

APPOINT A MEMBER OF YOUR TEAM TO INVESTIGATE

There is no reason why your staff nurses (both junior and senior) cannot investigate a complaint. It is good to be exposed to complaints early on in one's career. The fact that many complaints are due to poor communication and record keeping will help your staff appreciate the importance of such matters, particularly when their own investigation is hampered by poorly kept records.

For each complaint investigation, make sure enough time and support has been allocated. If necessary, go through the roster to ensure blocks of time can be freed up to carry out a thorough investigation. Ensure you are available to intervene if anyone is not co-operating. Don't leave them to struggle with people who refuse to make time to talk, or are being deliberately rude.

COLLATE THE WRITTEN INFORMATION

The investigation begins with the collation of relevant written documentation and meetings with the staff involved. This usually includes the following documents:

- The complainant's health records.
- Any trust-wide or local policies/procedures relevant to the complaint.
- Copies of relevant rosters or on-call rotas to identify who was on duty at the time.
- A copy of the original complaint and any other correspondence.

Relevant papers from the medical records may include medical and/or nursing progress sheets, consent forms, test request forms, GP referral letters, etc. Remember that physiotherapists and occupational therapists tend to keep separate case notes stored in their own departments. These may need to be located too. It's essential that you keep accurate notes of the investigation process in the form of a running log of events and findings. An example of an investigation progress sheet that could be used is outlined in Appendix 7.1.

MAINTAIN CONFIDENTIALITY

The complaints department will have informed the complainant that their records may be used and will have given them the option of refusing to allow this.

BOX 7.2: CALDICOTT PRINCIPLES

1. Justify the purpose.
2. Don't use patient identifiable information unless it is absolutely necessary.
3. Use the minimum necessary patient identifiable information.
4. Access to patient identifiable information should be on a strict need-to-know basis.
5. Everyone should be aware of their responsibilities.
6. Understand and comply with the law.

(Caldicott Committee 1997)

The Data Protection Act 1998 requires all processing of data to be 'fair and lawful' and all 'personal data to be protected against unauthorised or unlawful processing and against accidental loss, destruction or damage'. This means that while the investigator has the documents in their possession but is not using them directly, they should be kept in a locked drawer/filing cabinet and the office should be locked at all times when no one is there. The medical records should never be taken home under any circumstances.

As a health care professional, the investigator should follow their own professional code of confidentiality and the Caldicott principles (Box 7.2). You should also ensure they are aware of the appropriate NHS Code of Confidentiality which emphasises that patient information must remain confidential and seen only by those with direct involvement (Department of Health 2003, NHS Scotland 2008, NHS Wales 2005).

In addition, remember to ensure that any information about the complaint, including the original letter, is not filed in the medical or nursing notes. It must be kept separately. This also applies to verbal complaints. No notes of any complaints should be filed in patients' records.

INTERVIEW STAFF SENSITIVELY

Once all the documents have been obtained, the next stage is to identify the staff involved and make appointments to see them all. Remember that this is not a disciplinary process. The purpose of the meeting is simply to ascertain the facts. Formal statements are not required; however, it is wise for the investigator to write some notes of the meeting simply to remember the facts.

If the complaint is complex, you may decide to ask for witness statements. In that case, you must ensure that the individuals are informed of their rights to have a union representative, colleague or friend present. You should also ensure they are aware that their statements may be used if the complainant decides to take legal action at a later stage.

The appropriate records should be made available when meeting with individual members of staff, to help 'jog' their memory. The staff member also has a right to see the original letter of complaint. If any members of staff involved cannot remember the patient or what happened then they should say so; it is far better to admit this. In the final letter, you would simply say what you have concluded from the notes, but that the practitioner was unable to recall the details.

If at this stage you feel that the information cannot be assembled together within the time limit that was agreed, let the complaints department know. The complainant should also be contacted. You'll need to explain what the problem is and say when you will be able to give a full response. Remember: always 'under-promise and over-deliver'. If you think you will get the information and response out within the next few days, give them a date for 2 weeks' time. That way they will be impressed if they get the answer before the 2 weeks and it gives you some extra time to allow for unforeseen circumstances.

TIPS FOR CALLING OR MEETING WITH A COMPLAINANT

Simple complaints can often be settled with a phone call or a meeting with the patient, followed up with a written letter confirming what you have agreed. Inviting the complainant to meet and discuss the complaint can be a more successful option, particularly if they have lots of questions. Indeed, it is now encouraged as the first line of action on receipt of a written complaint. The complaints manager may or may not be involved, but it would be wise to use their expertise in such situations. Tips for holding a successful meeting follow.

PREPARATION

Arrange an appropriate venue

The meeting should be as informal as possible. It is preferable to use a non-clinical area, which is more familiar for the complainant. The complainant may bring other people with them for support so it is wise to book a good sized meeting room that can accommodate several people. Make sure there are chairs available in a waiting area outside. If there is more than one member of staff involved in the complaint and they need to be present, it is best to call them in one at a time when needed. To be in the same room with a group of health professionals can be quite intimidating for most people not used to the clinical environment.

Prepare a draft agenda with a timetable

This does not need to be formal but you will need some sort of structure to adhere to, otherwise you may end up going around in circles on the same subject with no conclusion. A list of the complaints may be all that is needed so that you can go through each one in turn. It is advisable to start by asking the complainant what they would like from the meeting.

Plan on the meeting lasting 1–1.5 hours at the most

If it goes over the hour, make sure the complainant is happy to go on and offer regular refreshments. Do not go over 1.5 hours unless absolutely necessary. By then everyone will be getting tired. Also they will probably have paid for the minimum 2 hours' parking time, which will cause added anxiety.

Make sure that all documents are available

Include case notes and copies of all correspondence pertaining to the complaint. You may need to refer to these during your discussions. You may also wish to share the contents with the complainant so it's a good idea to familiarise yourself with the contents and be prepared to explain any words or phrases which they may not understand.

Ensure there is someone else present to take notes

These will be used to form the basis of the follow-up letter, so will need to be detailed. If a nurse explained a procedure she undertook, for example, the notes would need to include that explanation. It would not be good enough for the complainant to read that 'the nurse explained the procedure'.

FACILITATION

Listen attentively

Make sure the complainant(s) knows they have your full attention. Turn the phone off and put up a 'Do not disturb' notice outside the door (including the date and time). Make brief notes as you go and let them see what you are writing. Don't write too much. You have a note-taker to do that for you. One of the reasons you write notes would be to reassure the complainant that you are taking them seriously.

Show them that you are listening through body language and regular prompts. Summarise what they are telling you as you go along. This not only shows them that you hear what they are saying, it also ensures that you are clear about it in your mind. For example:

- 'Just to clarify my understanding …'
- 'Would you mind just going over that bit again with me?'
- 'I have the impression that you feel … Is that right?'

Empathise

Let them know you understand what they are feeling or what they must have gone through. For example:

- 'I can see why you must be upset.'
- 'It must have been difficult for you.'
- 'I can understand why you felt so angry at the time.'

Don't suggest that what they are saying cannot be true or insinuate that they must be exaggerating, with phrases like:

- 'I can't believe she said it quite like that.'
- 'Are you sure that's what happened?'

This will only serve to aggravate the situation. It is advisable to neither agree nor disagree but remain neutral. Stick to empathising rather than sympathising. It will help focus the meeting on finding a solution rather than going through the problem over and over again.

Explain and apologise if appropriate

Explain why things have apparently gone wrong. If there are nursing records pertaining to the situation, let them see what has been written and explain any technical terms that they may not understand. Be open. If it is clear that a mistake has been made, then apologise and be sincere in that apology. They will want to know that you regret what happened and will take steps to ensure it does not happen again.

If there was no mistake and their complaint is unjustified then say so. However, it is often the case that poor communication somewhere along the way led them to this meeting. You will probably need at least to apologise that they were not better informed.

Make sure you have answered all their questions. Allow time for further questions. Don't be afraid of silences. Good use of silence gives people time to think and feel that they are still in control.

Agree a course of action

Once you have listened, empathised and/or apologised and answered all their questions, you need to agree a course of action:

- 'What would you like me to do now?'
- 'How would you like me to take this forward?'
- 'I suggest that from now on, we take the following steps to ensure it does not happen again ... would you be happy with this?'

If the complainant is satisfied, ensure the course of action agreed is achievable. If what the complainant is asking for is not realistic, then say so. It would be unrealistic, for example, if you are asked to dismiss a member of staff for speaking to them in a cursory manner. In this case you might say 'I cannot authorise what you are asking for. This member of staff has been formally spoken to. I do not condone her actions but am prepared to give her a second chance with close monitoring'.

Wrap up the meeting with a promise that you will look into things further if:

- what they are asking for is outside your remit
- they begin asking for too much
- they become angry and abusive
- further issues arise at the meeting that you were not previously aware of.

A few well-chosen words are called for, for example, 'It appears that there are further matters that need looking into, so you will need to give me some more time to look into this properly'.

Close the meeting appropriately

Close the meeting by summarising what has taken place and what you have agreed. Always explain what will happen next, that a letter will be sent confirming what has been discussed with any changes that you have agreed to implement. Give a timetable; don't say they will receive a letter by the end of the week unless you are absolutely certain that you can get it done by then. Remember to under-promise and over-deliver.

FOLLOW UP

Always do what you agreed to do. If you have promised to call the next day once you have made further enquires, then do so. Even if you do not have the information, call and say so, then arrange to call again when you have the information. Follow up is the most important stage in the complaints process. Too many complaints reach the Health Service Ombudsman because complainants do not receive that call/letter which they were promised. Failing to follow up agreed actions only serves to make a bad situation worse.

TIPS FOR WRITING A RESPONSE LETTER

Get the structure right

All letters should contain the following: a thank you (for raising the issue), an apology and/or a few words acknowledging the trouble it has caused them, an explanation of what happened, an outline of the action you are going to take, your contact details and an outline of what they can do next if still not satisfied.

If there are several subjects of complaint within one letter, prioritise the main complaint and address the minor points afterwards. Using subheadings for complaints with more than one aspect of care helps to keep it structured.

Represent your organisation

Always keep in mind that your reply is representing your organisation and the overall health care system. Saying negative things about the way it is managed is very unprofessional. It will result in the complainant losing their confidence in you. Don't hide behind the system or processes that are beyond your own control. If the issue is beyond your direct control, say what your organisation is doing about it or who is trying to rectify the 'system problem'.

You are speaking on behalf of your organisation. Complainants do not want to hear about any internal problems you may have with getting things done or poor communication between different departments. They are not interested if the broken toilet has not been mended because the facilities department have not responded to your numerous requests. If this is the case then you are simply showing them that you are not a good enough manager to be able to make things happen.

Write in 'the first person'

Don't try to present an anonymous face. Refer to yourself as 'I' and the complainant as 'you'. For example:

- *Anonymous response*: 'It is worrying to hear that the standard of care was not satisfactory.'
- *Personal response*: 'I am sorry to hear that you were not happy with the standard of care.'

Addressing the complainant as 'you' signifies to them that you are treating them as a real person and not just another complainant. Try not to use the term 'we' unless you are explaining organisational policy or decisions. The complainant is much more likely to believe and trust a single person. An anonymised 'we' represents a faceless organisation.

Add the personal touch

It is always best to put yourself in the complainant's shoes and think how you would feel if you went through a similar situation. Strike a personal note with them. Treat them as you would if you were speaking to a colleague. It helps to write as you speak, so they can almost hear the words. It's not just what you write, it's the way that you write it that makes the difference. The explanation and facts may be right but if they come across as formal and business-like, the complainant will not be satisfied.

Ensure your personality, professionalism and, above all, empathy shine through in the letter. The complainant will hopefully feel happy that everything that could be done is being done and that it's not just a standard bureaucratic response.

Another way to give your letter the personal touch is to write in the 'active' tense as opposed to the 'passive' tense. Consider the following:

● *Passive tense*: 'Please rest assured that action has been taken to rectify the situation.'
● *Active tense*: 'I can assure you that we are taking action to rectify the situation.'

The first sentence distances the writer and absolves any responsibility for the situation whereas, in the second example, the complainant can be reassured that someone is making sure something is being done. Taking a passive and distant tone is more 'business-like' but not appropriate when writing to a complainant.

Avoid using jargon

Keep it simple or at least explain technical terms where you use them. Most patients do not know the detailed hierarchical structure in health care. So using terms like health care support worker, physician, consultant, registrar or staff nurse should be avoided, or if you have to refer to these job titles then include an explanation about what they are. Try to stick to the generic terms 'doctor' or 'nurse'.

Use the same phrases you would use if you were talking to someone, not the official terms used in formal written communications. Use:

● 'about …' rather than 'with reference to …'
● 'I now know …' rather than 'I have since been informed …'
● 'because …' rather than 'due to the fact that …'
● 'I'm sorry' rather than 'please accept my apologies'.

Start with a thank you

First impressions count, so the way the letter starts is crucial. It sets the tone. This is why it is usually best to thank the complainant for the letter and for bringing the issue to your attention, followed by either an apology or a note of sympathy for their predicament. The opening paragraph should be kept short. Try not to use abbreviations such as 're:'. It depersonalises your reply immediately. Examples include:

- 'Thank for writing and bringing this issue to our attention.'
- 'Thank you for your letter about the problems you have had with …'

Apologise or empathise

Follow your opening lines with an apology or a few words of sympathy. Remember that an apology is not an admission of liability within the complaints process (NHSLA 2009). Empathising with the complainant does not equate to apologising. It shows that you are genuinely interested, supportive and understanding. Put yourself in their shoes and imagine how you would feel in the circumstances they describe. Show that you are making an effort to understand their point of view. If you have nothing to apologise for, then don't. You can say you understand without apologising, such as:

- 'I know how frustrating it is to be kept in the dark.'
- 'I can imagine this must have been very distressing for you.'

If you are sorry, say so, even if it is just because the letter is late:

- 'I am sorry for the delay in replying.'
- 'I am so sorry to hear of your recent loss.'
- 'I am extremely sorry this has happened.'

Explain the facts

Always give a full explanation of the facts but, again, make it personal. To say that 'this is what happened …' or 'these are the facts …' is too formal. Try the following examples:

- 'There seems to have been a major breakdown in communication in your case.'
- 'Unfortunately, it seems that the doctor forgot to tell the nurse he had prescribed the tablets to be given that night. The nurse had already given your father his tablets for the evening and so did not look at his chart again until the morning by which time it was too late.'

Outline what you have done or are going to do

Outlining what you are going to do about the situation is the main part of the letter. The complainant needs to be reassured that something is going to be done as a result of their complaint. They need to know that their letter is being taken seriously. Here are some examples of how to begin this section:

- 'This has highlighted a gap in our system, so what I am going to do is …'
- 'As a direct result of your complaint, we have/will …'
- 'I can assure you that in order to reduce the risk of this happening again, I have decided to …'

Give your contact details

Always finish by giving your contact details. A few extra words at this stage can help to make it feel more genuine. Here are some examples to stimulate your thoughts (and again to save you time):

- 'We will do everything possible to reduce the risk of this happening again.'
- 'Thank you again for bringing this to our attention.'
- 'I am sorry that we cannot be more helpful on this occasion, but hope you have been reassured that …'
- 'I hope this explains the position, but if you have any other queries, please feel free to contact me.'

These are just some examples to stimulate your own thinking. It is worth building up a series of stock phrases for the future when you have to write something at short notice during a busy period.

Remember it doesn't take much to add the personal touch. Rather than write the usual 'please do not hesitate to contact me', the following will have a far better effect: 'I do hope this answers your questions, but should there be anything else you need to know I'll be happy to discuss it further if you call me at … Alternatively, you can call our Patient Experience Team at …'.

Giving them your direct contact details will hopefully ensure that any further issues can be solved through a telephone call. It is far better to do this than end up receiving another letter to which you have to compile yet another response.

Check the layout is easy to read

Once you have written the response letter, spend some time on making it look good and easier to read. Ensure the following:

- All paragraphs should be wider than they are long.
- Use bullet points where you can to break up the text.
- Use subheadings if more than one complaint is incorporated.
- Have one idea per paragraph and keep sentences short.

Confirm the final letter (or report) with all staff involved

The final letter or report must be checked and agreed by *all* staff involved in the complaint investigation to ensure it is factually correct. Confirm that all points raised in the initial letter have been answered, and the main one is answered first.

Once all those involved have agreed that it is a fair and accurate account of what actually happened, return your final response to the complaints department. Never send a response letter straight to the complainant. Most complaints procedures require that either the chief executive signs all response letters or a cover letter by the chief executive is included. The complaints team will ensure that this is done. They will also check through your letter to ensure it complies with various organisational procedures. For the more complex complaints (such as those involving other departments), you may only be required to send the results of your investigation to the complaints team and someone within the department will write the response from your report.

INVESTIGATE INCIDENTS APPROPRIATELY

Observe the trends from your incident forms and work closely with your team to reduce the risk of further incidents of the same nature happening again. Don't wait to be told what your main issues are from the risk management or clinical governance lead.

INCIDENT FORMS

Make your team aware that sending off an incident form does not absolve them of the responsibility of ensuring that something is done. Also, remember that completing an incident form does not equate to an admission of liability. The purpose of incident reporting is to support you and your team to learn from incidents, not to blame. Incident reports should concentrate on what happened and why, not who. The exceptions to this rule are:

- cases of gross negligence
- if someone has been malicious, deliberately negligent or carried out a criminal act
- where there have been similar incidents and someone's actions have continued despite remedial actions being undertaken.

Encourage your staff to complete incident forms thoroughly and to think carefully about their responsibilities following an incident. Writing an incident form does not absolve that member of staff from responsibility. In the section entitled 'Action taken', it is not acceptable to only write that someone senior has been informed. They must be encouraged to write what specific action they have taken themselves. For example, if an incident form is completed because reduced staffing levels are considered unsafe, the person-in-charge must outline all the steps they have taken to ensure the patients are safe, not just who they have informed. They should outline what priorities they have made with the team, and what work will be left undone (e.g. making beds, administration, audits, meetings, ward rounds) in order to maintain patient safety

Copies of all incident forms are simply logged and it is the role of your line manager or matron to ensure they are reviewed across the directorate on a regular basis to reduce the risk of further incidents. Take the initiative and do this first with your team before waiting to be told what to do. It will make your life a lot easier in the long term.

SERIOUS INCIDENTS REQUIRING INVESTIGATION (SIRIs)

If the incident constitutes a SIRI, your organisational policy will outline the steps you should follow regarding communications and dealing with the actual incident. A SIRI is an incident that:

- has resulted in serious harm or death
- is of major public or media concern
- involves allegations of abuse
- threatens your organisation's ability to deliver health care
- is one of the 'never events' (see Box 7.3).

BOX 7.3: THE NEVER EVENTS LIST

A 'never event' is a serious but preventable incident that should not occur with the appropriate systems in place. All 'never events' have to be reported both to the commissioners and the CQC in England, and should be subject to a root cause analysis investigation.

1. Wrong site surgery.
2. Wrong implant/prosthesis.
3. Retained foreign object post-operation.
4. Wrongly prepared high-risk injectable medication.
5. Maladministration of potassium-containing solutions.
6. Wrong route administration of chemotherapy.
7. Wrong route administration of oral/enteral treatment.
8. Intravenous administration of epidural medication.
9. Maladministration of insulin.
10. Overdose of midazolam during conscious sedation.
11. Opioid overdose of an opioid-naïve patient.
12. Inappropriate administration of daily oral methotrexate.
13. Suicide using non-collapsible rails.
14. Escape of a transferred prisoner (from medium or high secure mental health services).
15. Falls from unrestricted windows.
16. Entrapment in bedrails.
17. Transfusion of ABO-incompatible blood components.
18. Transplantation of ABO- or HLA-incompatible organs.
19. Misplaced naso- or orogastric tubes.
20. Wrong gas administered.
21. Failure to monitor and respond to oxygen saturation.
22. Air embolism.
23. Misidentification of patients.
24. Severe scalding of patients.
25. Maternal death due to post-partum haemorrhage after elective caesarean section.

(Department of Health 2011)

If you are unsure, it is best to report it as a potential SIRI. A serious incident still warrants the completion of an incident form but, in addition, you should gather any relevant information, photocopy any relevant clinical notes, keep faulty equipment and gather information from witnesses within 24 hours of the incident. This information will form the basis of further investigations. You should ensure that your line manager is informed immediately as well as the patient's consultant. The patient and their relatives should also be informed but do not attempt to do this by yourself if you feel at all unsure. You should have specific training on communicating with patients and relatives following serious incidents.

An investigation team is usually nominated to undertake a further review in the case of confirmed SIRIs. You may be nominated to assist with the investigation and writing of the report. This is usually carried out using the root cause analysis approach.

ROOT CAUSE ANALYSIS

The root cause analysis approach focuses on identifying the sequence of events and allowing the root cause of the incident to emerge. A serious incident is often not just the result of human error but a chain of events that led to the human error.

The investigation should result in recommendations for improving systems and processes to prevent the risk of a similar human error occurring again.

A senior person will be appointed to take the lead in the investigation and will gather a small team of individuals to assist. They will go through the following steps:

1. Data collection: this involves visiting the area where the incident took place, collecting information including the original incident report and any related policies, gathering statements and meeting witnesses.
2. Putting all the data in chronological order: some sort of timeline will be produced outlining what happened and when, and perhaps who was doing what at certain times.
3. Review meetings: a series of meetings will be held with the investigating team and any other relevant professionals (including those involved in the incident) to explore the data, using specific tools to help them pinpoint exactly what contributing factors led to the incident. The main contributing factors will then be explored in further depth to determine their root causes. A number of tools can be used; one commonly used tool is the 'five whys' (see Fig. 7.1).
4. Report: the lead investigator will put together a report detailing the investigative process, the identified root causes of the incident and recommendations for changes to be put in place to reduce the risk of further similar incidents.

If you or any of your staff were involved in the incident, you should be given the opportunity to review and agree the contents of the final report. Remember that this report is an analysis of the systems which were at fault, not the people involved. And like all reports, it should present the facts, not opinions, and demonstrate that the incident has been thoroughly and fairly investigated. It is not a tool with which to punish people. The whole point of incident investigations is to learn from them. If a mistake is made, it is usually an 'honest human error'. The only human errors that are punishable are those that can be defined as 'dishonest'.

If it is found during the investigation that a health professional has been dishonest in any way or has deliberately flouted protocols without any justification, then a different procedure will be used, usually the disciplinary policy (see p. 72). The individual concerned will be advised to contact their trade union representative. However, in the vast majority of cases, human error is caused by one or more system faults. There is no point in punishing people for honest errors. In fact, some would argue that it is dangerous to do so because it will only serve to stop us from being able to learn from the errors (Vincent 2010).

CONTRIBUTING TO INCIDENT INVESTIGATION REPORTS

As a ward manager, you will probably not be required to write a full incident investigation report unless you have received full training and are appointed as a lead investigator. However, you may be asked to contribute some sections towards the overall report, so it is worth being aware of what is involved. There are lots of things to consider. For example, the patient or their relatives have the right to read the report, so you have to be sensitive to their feelings.

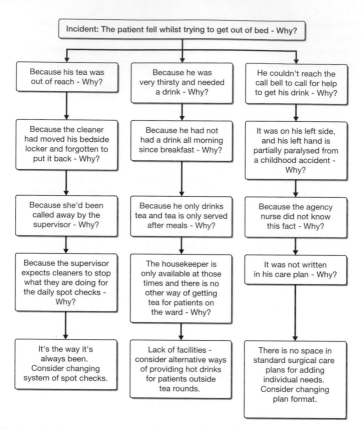

Fig. 7.1 Five whys tool. An example of how it can be used for getting to the root cause of incidents.

Incident investigation reports differ enormously from disciplinary investigation reports, because they focus on system faults (that may or may not cause human error) whereas disciplinary reports focus on allegations of human misconduct or deliberate harm. This means that the staff involved should not be identified by name. Even the patient involved should be given a pseudonym, unless they and/or their relatives express a preference for their real name to be used. The report should also be written objectively in the third person.

The National Reporting and Learning Service (NRLS) for England and Wales produced an excellent guide to investigation report writing following root cause analysis of patient safety incidents (NRLS 2008) which is a must to read if you are ever involved in an SIRI or any other root cause analysis incident investigation. It recommends the following headings be used:

- An executive summary.
- A description of the incident and its consequences.
- Pre-investigation risk assessment.
- Background and context of the incident.
- Terms of reference.
- The investigation team.
- The scope and level of the investigation.
- The investigation type, process and methods used.
- Involvement and support of the patient, relatives and carers.
- Involvement and support of staff involved in the incident.
- Information and evidence gathered.
- Chronology of events leading up to the incident.
- Detection of incident.
- Notable practice within the case.
- Care and service delivery problems.
- Contributory factors.
- Root causes.
- Lessons learned.
- Recommendations.
- Arrangements for shared learning.
- Distribution list.
- Appendices.

Once an investigative incident report is finished you must ensure that you, and anyone else in your team who was involved in the incident, have the opportunity to read it and check for inaccuracies. And later, it's advisable to obtain a copy of the report for the rest of your team to read and discuss at one of your team meetings. This ensures that all learn from the incident, both from the recommendations and also by seeing first hand that incident investigation reports are all about learning and not punishing individuals involved. All too often, staff do not get to read the report and just get 'told' the actions that they have to take from now on, creating both resentment and a reluctance to report any future serious incidents.

MAKE IMPROVEMENTS

DISCUSS EVERYTHING WITH YOUR TEAM

Discussing incidents and complaints regularly with your team is a good way of showing them that you are listening and learning and willing to make changes. It reduces the risk of staff saying 'What's the use of filling in all these incident forms if no one ever reads them or does anything about them?' If you are willing to make improvements in practice, particularly as a result of incident reports, your staff will feel more encouraged to report them. The more incidents that are reported, the safer your working practices will be. The more you discuss patient complaints, the less your staff will feel threatened by complaint investigations and more open to learning from them.

Unfortunately, more often than not, the time that is spent on investigating and compiling responses and reports can exceed that which is spent on making the actual improvements. Despite national policies being continually reviewed in order to simplify the processes and make them more customer and safety focused, many organisations have a tendency to bureaucratise such matters at a local level. Try and ensure that you do not allow yourself to get caught up in this bureaucracy and so lose sight of the whole purpose of the procedure.

Complaints provide you with important information and feedback about the experiences of patients on your ward. Incident reporting provides you with important information on safety issues. You must ensure that lessons are learned from both. Make them a regular item on your team meeting agenda.

FOLLOW UP WITH ACTION

Follow up all the actions at each meeting to ensure the issues raised previously are not overshadowed by the newer ones. A continuous plan of action from complaints and incidents should be maintained and updated regularly. This will ensure your team view them as an opportunity to improve services and make changes, rather than as a hassle. There is nothing worse than managers who continually procrastinate about the number of complaints and incidents they have to deal with.

DISSEMINATE THE LEARNING

Notice board displaying the learning from complaints

Getting no complaints at all does not mean you have a better service; it probably means the patients either don't know how to complain, are worried that you might take offence or that their future care may be affected. It is important that you state in your ward leaflet or information board that you welcome comments as a way of finding out what your patients really think.

Having a comment card system on your ward with a notice-board for staff, patients and their relatives displaying examples of responses is the practice of a progressive ward manager (see p. 94). It helps reduce the number of complaints but enables you to continue getting feedback. Without continuous comments and complaints, you can never be sure that the service you provide is truly meeting the patients' needs. You can put up extracts of written complaints (anonymised) and associated responses so that other patients and users of the service can see that you listen to their concerns and are actually doing something about it.

Notice board displaying the learning from incidents

This board is probably best displayed in your staff room. Like the comments/complaints notice board, it would be good to display the outcome of incident investigations but, more importantly, the actions that you have agreed to take with the team. The problem with running a department 24 hours a day, 7 days a week is that you cannot have all the team present at your team meetings. Displaying the results of your regular reviews and agreed action plans on a staff notice board will again encourage staff to be more open when reporting incidents and encouraged to see that they are being heard (and not punished).

Other wards and departments

Try to ensure that you are discussing the complaints and incidents across both your directorate and your organisation. Keep your matron informed so that they in turn can discuss the issues raised with their colleagues. Raise the issues for discussion at your ward sisters' meetings. Many ward managers work in isolation and assume that what they are doing or experiencing is happening in other parts of the hospital. That is often not the case. It has been known for certain incidents to be investigated in one part of an organisation but in another part, the same incidents may not even have been identified as requiring an incident report.

Some areas may not be so open in discussing their incidents and therefore staff may not report them because of concerns about the increased workload or fear of disciplinary action. You may be progressive in investigating and learning from complaints and incidents, but that will not necessarily be the case for all areas. Don't let it put you off sharing your practice with others, and thus hopefully stimulating them to share their practice with you too.

ACTION POINTS

- Ensure you are familiar with the origin of all quality indicators so that you can understand their significance and prioritise if necessary.
- Ensure that you and your staff receive appropriate training and support in handling complaints and incidents according to your local policy.
- If there is anything you are unsure about, get help early on from your line manager, complaints manager or risk manager. Better still, incorporate the complaints and risk managers into your network before you have to call on their services.
- Make sure the complaints or incident investigation process is halted if you suspect negligence, misconduct, a crime has been committed or anything that you feel requires a formal managerial investigation.
- If you don't have one already, put up an information board in your ward with comment cards and extracts of comments (anonymised) with responses, and an incident information board in your staff office.
- Inform and involve your team in all complaint and incident investigations and resulting action plans, preferably by having it on the agenda of all regular team meetings.

References

Armstrong, D., 2010. The power of apology. Focus. NHS Education for Scotland. Online. Available: http://www.nes.scot.nhs.uk/media/6338/Apology%20Spring%20Focus%202010.pdf Feb 2012.

Caldicott Committee, 1997. Report on the review of patient-identifiable information. Department of Health, London.

Care Quality Commission, 2010. Essential standards of quality and safety. Guidance about compliance. Online. Available: http://www.cqc.org.uk/guidanceforprofessionals/nhstrusts/complyingwiththeregulations/guidanceaboutcompliance.cfm Feb 2012.

Data Protection Act. 1998. HMSO, London. Online. Available: http://www.opsi.gov.uk/acts/acts1998/19980029.htm Feb 2012.

Department of Health, 2003. Confidentiality: NHS code of practice. Online. Available: http://www.dh.gov.uk/assetRoot/04/06/92/54/04069254.pdf Feb 2012.

Department of Health, 2010. Cycle of continuous improvement and development. Online. Available: http://www.dh.gov.uk/en/Aboutus/Chiefprofessionalofficers/Chiefnursingofficer/Energiseforexcellence/imagemap/DH_120962 Feb 2012.

Department of Health, 2011. The 'never events' list 2011/2012. Online. Available: http://www.dh.gov.uk/prod_consum_dh/groups/dh_digitalassets/documents/digitalasset/dh_124580.pdf Feb 2012.

National Patient Safety Agency, 2009. Being open: supporting information: patient safety alert NPSA/2009/PSA003. Online. Available: http://www.nrls.npsa.nhs.uk/beingopen/ Feb 2012.

National Reporting and Learning Service, 2008. Guide to investigation report writing following Root Cause Analysis of patient safety incidents. Online. Available: http://www.nrls.npsa.nhs.uk/resources Feb 2012.

NHS Information Centre, 2011. Indicators for quality improvement. Online. Available: https://mqi.ic.nhs.uk/ Feb 2012.

NHS Litigation Authority, 2009. Letter to chief executives and finance directors, all NHS bodies: apologies and explanations. Online. Available: http://www.nhsla.com/NR/rdonlyres/00F14BA6-0621-4A23-B885-FA18326FF745/0/ApologiesandExplanations.pdf Feb 2012.

NHS Scotland, 2008. NHS code of practice on protecting patient confidentiality. Scottish Executive. Online. Available: http://www.elib.scot.nhs.uk/SharedSpace/ig/Uploads/2008/Oct/20081002150659_6074NHSCode.pdf Feb 2012.

NHS Wales, Social Services Inspectorate for Wales and Welsh Assembly Government, 2005. Confidentiality: code of practice for health and social care in Wales. Online. Available: http://www.wales.nhs.uk/sites3/Documents/783/Confidentiality%20CodeofPractice.pdf Feb 2012.

Parliamentary and Health Service Ombudsman, 2010. Listening and learning: the Ombudsman's review of complaint handling by the NHS in England 2009–10. The Stationery Office, London. Online. Available: http://nhsreport.ombudsman.org.uk/.

Vincent, C., 2010. Patient safety. Wiley-Blackwell, Sussex.

EXAMPLE OF PROGRESS SHEET FOR A COMPLAINT INVESTIGATION

Action	Date completed and any comments
1. Complaint letter received	
2. Contact complainant to clarify their expectations or any unclear issues	
3. Appoint member of team (if appropriate)	
4. Meet with appointed member of team: – Agree issues to be investigated – Agree time out in diary to devote to investigation	
5. Investigator: – Locate patient's notes – Find further relevant documents – Identify and arrange to see staff involved	
6. Investigator: – Meet staff involved – Find out what happened and why	
7. Compile response letter or report	
8. Check final response/report with all staff involved	
9. Send final response/report to complaints department	
10. Return patient notes to medical records department	
11. Lock away the file in a safe and secure place	

CHAPTER 8

INSTIGATE A ROLLING RECRUITMENT PROGRAMME

If you could have all your vacancies filled at all times with the right staff with the right skills, wouldn't life be so much easier? Unfortunately this rarely seems to happen in real life, but you can go some way toward making things a lot easier for yourself if you concentrate on the recruitment process all the time, even when all your vacancies are filled. Nurses rarely stay in one post throughout their career. Having a fairly high turnover of staff seems to be the norm.

Change can be a good thing, however, and it's good for staff to regularly have new people join, with different skills to offer. It prevents them from becoming too comfortable and set in their ways. It also helps you to continually review and change your staffing establishment according to the needs of your unit. Make sure you are always one step ahead so that when a person resigns you will be able to replace them quickly without causing too much disruption.

REVIEW THE POST WITH THE PERSON WHO IS LEAVING

Before you even begin thoughts of advertising and filling a forthcoming vacancy, you should first review the role with the person who is leaving.

ESTABLISH WHY THEY ARE LEAVING

Staff may leave your team for promotion or to gain further experience. It could also be for personal reasons such as moving house or wanting to spend more time with children. You should be concerned if any members of staff are leaving for better working conditions, better hours or because of any problems at work. Take note of why they are leaving, and do something to ensure the next candidate will not feel the same way.

Don't leave exit interviews to the human resources (HR) department. All members of staff have a right to fill in an anonymous exit questionnaire when they leave, but you need feedback too. You don't need them to fill in any forms; just ask them. Remember though that employees have the right to refuse an exit interview. They should always be voluntary.

When you ask why someone is leaving, aim to ensure the person talks a lot more than you do. Spend most of the time listening and taking notes (even if you do not agree). Ask questions such as the following:

1. Are there any other reasons for leaving?
2. What could we do/have done to persuade you to stay?
3. What have you enjoyed or found satisfying about working here?
4. What aspects of work didn't you like or found difficult or frustrating?
5. Is there any more training and development you would have benefited from?
6. Is there anything that could be improved in the ward which would make things better from your point of view?
7. What is it about your next job that makes it more attractive than this one?

ESTABLISH IF THE JOB DESCRIPTION IS STILL APPROPRIATE

Review the job description with them. Has it changed in any way? If the remit has grown to include other responsibilities such as a vital link nurse role, first ask any of your other staff if they would like to take it on. If not, consider adding it to the job description. If, for example, the person is a link nurse for diabetes and it is a much needed role on the ward, then think about recruiting someone who has, or is willing to develop, those skills. Add it to the job description before you advertise.

The job could have changed so much that the person leaving may say it needs someone more senior with specialist experience or perhaps even someone who does not need the skills of a registered nurse any more. If this is the case, review this idea with the rest of the team. You may all come to the decision that it would be beneficial to replace this person with someone requiring entirely different skills from another pay band. It is advisable in such cases to meet with your finance manager and line manager to go through what you would need to do to change the post and pay band but remain within budget.

Changing the job and associated pay band

You cannot change your budgeted 'establishment' immediately because it has to be done through the business planning process. However, you do not have to match the budgeted establishment exactly. You can recruit a band 5 nurse into a health care assistant (HCA) post, for example, but only if you consult with your finance advisor and line manager first, to make sure that at the end of the year you will not go over budget in order to do so. The finance advisor will work it out for you, taking other issues into consideration such as:

- part-time staff in full-time posts
- staff who are on maternity leave
- staff on long-term sick leave
- current use of agency and bank staff.

Try and think 'outside the box'. There is no reason why you cannot redesign the job into one that suits your ward. You may, for example, like to devise a new role such as an HCA who can also take on part-time ward receptionist duties. This could help enormously at times when your current ward receptionist is on annual leave or off sick.

REVIEW THE JOB DESCRIPTION AND PERSON SPECIFICATION

The job description may need completely rewriting or just a few minor changes. Do this together with the person who is leaving the job. Your HR advisor will advise you on what you can and cannot do with the job description according to your organisation's policies and procedures.

Redesigning roles when a member of staff leaves helps to replace outdated jobs and allows your remaining team to progress by taking on different responsibilities. You can design jobs around the patient and changing workloads rather than the other way around. It is not a difficult thing to do. The key is to ensure you involve the right people, i.e. your finance advisor, your HR advisor and your line manager.

TAKE ACTION IF THE POST IS FROZEN OR REMOVED

Unfortunately, it is common nowadays for ward managers to be prevented from replacing staff members when they leave. If your budget is cut back like this, then you need to take action to prevent the rest of your team from becoming overworked. Take some time to work out exactly what it will mean for your team. One less member of staff means that five shifts per week (i.e. 5 out of 21 shifts) will have one less person. You therefore have to make adjustments to your roster. Choose which shifts will have one less member of staff. For example, in order to maintain safety, you could cut one person from each weekend shift. However, you must not 'burn out' the rest of the staff working at weekends, so you would need to agree with your team which aspects of work will no longer get done at weekends. Patient safety and care are essential, so generally it could be the paperwork such as audits (performance indicators, etc.) that will not get done. Agree this with your managers – in writing. If they won't agree, then work together with them to identify something else (equivalent to the work of one member of staff per shift) that will not get done.

If you are already busy on every shift, then you cannot achieve the same amount of work with one less staff member. Find more efficient ways of working with the staff you have. Usually this means that you have to agree certain aspects of work will no longer get done or will get done in a different way. Do not just cope and allow your team to work extra unpaid hours to cover up for short-staffing. It contravenes the Health and Safety Executive (HSE) guidelines on managers' responsibility for balancing job demands with the availability of staff (HSE 2011).

WRITE GOOD ADVERTS AND APPLICATION PACKAGES

Don't leave the writing of your job adverts and application packages to your HR department. State exactly what you want in the advert and give them the material for your application packages. List what you want to be sent out to each prospective candidate.

PUT IN EXTRA EFFORT

Don't leave anything to chance. The recruitment teams in HR departments have a huge remit. They have to oversee the recruitment for all personnel within your organisation. Don't expect them to give you special treatment. They will send out standard application packages and do not usually have the capacity to make up specific ones for your ward. So send them additional information to add to your application packages. Don't approach it with the attitude 'it's not my job'. That will get you nowhere. If you really want to recruit the right staff, then you have to put in the effort, whether it's your job or not.

WRITING THE ADVERT

Involve your whole team in devising what to put in the job advert. Include the person who is leaving. They are the ones who browse through the job adverts regularly. Ask them which adverts are the ones which catch their attention. Ask them which parts of the job would be the most attractive for new staff. Getting that advert right is crucial. Most advertising is now carried out online through sites such as 'NHS Jobs' which means prospective candidates get to see only the first four lines of the advert at a glance, so concentrate on making these the most eye-catching.

Make the closing date for 3–4 weeks' time. If you give only 2 weeks, you are ruling out all potential candidates who are on annual leave at the time of the advert. Put the interview date on the advert too. It quickens up the process. The interview date could then be around 2 weeks after the closing date. Having the interview date on the advert gives the candidate plenty of time to prepare. Waiting until you shortlist candidates before you decide on an interview date only serves to delay the process unnecessarily. You will also have a number of candidates who will not be able to attend, thus prolonging the process even further by having to set a second date. Make things easier and straightforward for you and the candidate by putting both the closing date and interview date on the advert in the first place.

Remember to attach the revised job description and person specification when you send the final advert to your HR recruitment department.

APPLICATION PACKAGES

When the HR team receives enquiries, all they are required to do is send out a copy of the job description and person specification. Some send out information about your organisation too. If you really want to interest potential candidates, give your HR department further information about your ward.

Again, ask your team what they think would be good to include in the application package. A group of people are a lot more creative than one or two on their own. Possible options include:

- a photograph of your team, happy and smiling
- a copy of your team's annual plan of goals/objectives
- some quotes from your staff saying what is good about working on your ward
- an explanation of your method of working, e.g. team or primary nursing, and perhaps even a sample of your roster showing how you organise yourselves and to prove that you do not expect them to work awful shift patterns.

Be careful not to give the impression that the ward is better than it is. The last thing you need is to recruit people under false pretences; they won't stay long. Disillusioned newcomers will disillusion your team.

SHORTLIST AND ARRANGE INTERVIEWS PROPERLY

Most health care organisations now have a database of professionals who have been removed from the register or any former employees or agency staff who should not be employed with you again. Before you shortlist the candidates, make sure that all the names have been checked against this database.

TIPS FOR SHORTLISTING

1. *Shortlist within 5 days of the closing date.* Make sure you block out some time for this in your diary when you put in the advert.
2. *Shortlist with another person from your team.* Don't shortlist on your own. At least one of the people involved in the shortlisting needs to be on the interview panel.
3. *Base the shortlisting on the person specification.* Check that the candidates meet all the 'essential' criteria. The 'desirable' criteria need only be used when a particularly large number of candidates meet the 'essential' criteria.
4. *Keep a note of the reasons for selection and rejection of all candidates* which confirms that the same criteria were used for all candidates. Send a copy to the HR department, so that they can deal with any follow up requests for information from rejected candidates. It will also help should there be any complaints or allegations of discrimination.
5. *Get the results of the shortlisting over to your recruitment department as soon as possible.* It is in your interests to show prospective candidates that this is a good place to work. Receiving an interview letter with only a few days to spare does not create a good impression.
6. *Try to ensure that requests for references are sent out at the shortlisting stage.* This will prevent any delays in offering the post to the successful candidate. Most application forms give the individual the option to not have references taken up until after the interview, so you need to make sure that you do not breach the individual's stated wishes.

PREPARE FOR THE INTERVIEWS

You will already have your interview date set from the advertising stage. You need a minimum of two people.

At least one of the interviewers should have had formal training in recruitment and selection, which includes information on the equal opportunity aspects of recruitment and the relevant legislation. Avoid having any more than three people on the interview panel as it can be intimidating to candidates at this level.

Holding interviews in your ward or department office is a good idea so long as you have the space and can guarantee there will be no interruptions. Make sure there is an allocated area outside the room where candidates can wait. The candidates will feel at ease because it is an environment they are used to. It can be daunting for clinical staff to enter formal office environments. They are unfamiliar places for health care professionals, particularly the more junior ones, and may serve to make them more nervous.

Remember also that there are obligations under the Single Equality Act 2010 to ensure that disabled applicants (or those that are carers or associated with someone who is disabled) are not discriminated against or disadvantaged in any way (see www.equalities.gov.uk). The HR team should have asked in the interview offer letter if individuals require any special assistance on that day. You should check before the interview if anyone has requested such assistance.

PREPARE YOUR TEAM FOR THE INTERVIEWS

Check the roster to ensure you have good 'numbers' on at the time of interviews and ensure all your staff are aware to be prepared for the arrival of prospective candidates. Agree with your team what they should do to greet them when they arrive. Everyone needs to create a good impression. Your staff on that shift should:

- keep a look out for the interviewees arriving
- greet them warmly with a welcoming smile
- show them where they can wait
- inform them where the nearest toilets are
- offer them a drink
- offer to show them around the ward while they are waiting.

All this serves to confirm that your ward is a good one to work where all the staff are nice and friendly. Even if you do not offer the candidate a post, they will go away thinking what a nice place it is and tell all their friends and colleagues, who will tell their friends and colleagues. Word spreads quickly among health care staff. You don't want a disgruntled candidate telling everyone they wouldn't have taken the job anyway because it didn't look like a good place to work.

GET THE BEST OUT OF THE INTERVIEW PROCESS

Each candidate should leave feeling they have been welcomed, treated fairly and given every opportunity to demonstrate their suitability for the job.

PREPARING THE QUESTIONS

Prepare the interview questions in advance. Questions should be tailored to the person specification. In other words, you want to find out how the candidate meets the desirable criteria. You have already determined the essential criteria from the application form. Questions should also be included to find out:

- why they have applied for this job
- what qualities they can bring to the team
- their level of competence in practice.

You can also ask questions to get them to expand on what they have written on the application form. What you must not include are any questions about the candidates' personal circumstances such as how they organise their childcare or whether they are married or in a relationship.

Be consistent

You should ask the same set of questions to each candidate. This is to ensure they all have the same opportunities to present the best of themselves. It does not mean you have to keep rigidly to the wording of each question. You can vary them according to the answers given. There is also nothing wrong with asking further probing questions to expand on the answer(s) given.

Try and stick to open questions to encourage the candidate to talk freely. The aim is to ensure the candidate does most of the talking. Avoid leading questions or closed questions. Encourage them to give their own answer, not the answer that you would like to be given.

ASSESSMENT OF PRACTICAL SKILLS

It is very difficult to assess a candidate's practical competence in an interview. Presentations serve mainly to assess their presentation skills. One of the ways you can assess their practical skills is to include a set of questions based on scenarios:

- 'What action would you take if ...?'
- 'How would you deal with a situation where ...?'
- 'If X happened, what would you do?'

Another good way of eliciting information from candidates is to get them to quantify their experience, using questions like:

- 'How many times have you ...?'
- 'What is your experience to date regarding ...?'

The use of some sort of written test can help you to assess the practical aspects too. Present them with a couple of scenarios and ask them to write down what they would do. You could give them a situation where they have to prioritise as they would if they were in charge of a shift. Ask them to write down their rationale for each action.

If you decide to include a written assessment, you must do the following:

1. Let the HR department know at the short-listing stage, so they can inform the candidates in the letter inviting them for interview.
2. Allow for the extra time required in the interview timetable.
3. Organise a separate quiet room where candidates can undertake the exercise undisturbed.
4. Make sure that the questions relate specifically to criteria outlined in the person specification.

Whatever method you use for assessment and interviewing, it is essential to set up a scoring system such as marks out of five for each question. Each interviewer will then score the person separately. These can assist with the final decision.

PREPARE THE ENVIRONMENT AND INTERVIEWERS

Tidy up the room if needed. Set out the chairs, preferably so that you can see the clock on the wall behind the interviewee. Continuously looking at your wristwatch during the interview is disconcerting for the candidate. Sit in the candidate's chair to see if it is a comfortable distance away from the interviewers' chairs and there are no diversions such as glaring sunlight from the window.

Divert the phones and any pagers, and ensure everyone turns off their mobile phones. Put a very big notice on the door saying 'Interviews in Progress' with the date and time. Include the time when you will be finishing.

THE ROLE OF THE CHAIRPERSON IN INTERVIEWS

Before you begin the interviews, identify which one of you will chair the process. Normally it would be you, but your junior staff members have to gain the experience some time and it is best they do it at a time when they can receive support and guidance from a more experienced interviewer. The role of the chair is to:

1. Introduce yourself and the other interviewers.
2. Settle the candidate by using small talk such as 'Did you find your way alright?'
3. Explain the interview plan and that you will be taking notes throughout the process.
4. Give some background information about your ward.
5. Facilitate the flow of questions.
6. Allow silences to ensure the candidate gets a chance to consider their thoughts before answering.
7. Ensure that the candidate does most of the speaking.
8. Keep to the timeframe.
9. Ask if the candidate has any questions at the end.
10. Ensure they give you the appropriate documents, e.g. occupational health form, ID such as passport, etc. (HR will advise you beforehand as to what is required).
11. Thank the candidate for attending.
12. Inform the candidate what will happen next, and when you will be making the decision.

FOLLOW UP ALL CANDIDATES PERSONALLY

Make your choice and write up your notes immediately after interview. Keep all your notes and scoring results from the interviews. They help when feeding back to candidates, especially if you are required to feedback a few weeks or even months after the interview. Make sure the records are accurate and objective with no reference to personal opinions. Under data protection laws, candidates have a right to see these notes after the interview if they so wish.

Most people prefer to call the candidates personally. Don't promise to call them that evening. Remember: 'under-promise and over-deliver'. It will cause you undue hassle if you say you will call them that evening then find that you are unable to make a final decision for some reason. Give yourself at least a day's grace, in case of any problems. Always caveat any verbal offers with them being subject to satisfactory checks (e.g. Criminal Records Bureau clearance).

Don't offer the job before receiving the references. It will cause you immense problems if you receive unsatisfactory references after offering the job. The references usually just confirm that you have made a good decision, but if they do not you will need to follow them up. That takes time. You can telephone the referees if you have not received a written reference. You can ask them to send you a fax or e-mail. A detailed record of the call including the date, time and the person you spoke to may suffice.

CALLING UNSUCCESSFUL CANDIDATES

Nobody likes to be the bearer of bad news. However, it is a nice gesture to call the unsuccessful candidates as soon as possible after the interviews, rather than let them wait for the official letter. Handle the situation by turning it into a positive experience:

1. Begin by telling the candidate they were unsuccessful.
2. Follow this immediately by telling them what they did well and which parts impressed you.
3. Then, tell them the reason why they did not get the job. Be precise but do not dwell on this part. Stick to one or two comments then follow it up by offering further feedback at a later date should they want it.

Once the candidate is told that they have been unsuccessful, they are not usually in the mood to have a discussion about what they did wrong. However, they may want further feedback at a later date. Offer this service and make sure you are genuine in your offer. Tell them you have made lots of notes and are more than willing to spend time giving them further information about what they can do to improve next time. Remember that your aim is to make sure that everyone sees your ward in a positive light, even unsuccessful job applicants.

FOLLOW UP PROMISING BUT UNSUCCESSFUL CANDIDATES

If you only have one vacancy but two or three really good candidates, don't just take one and say goodbye to the rest. Speak to your colleagues. Do they have any vacancies? Does your HR team know of any other vacancies which you think the candidates may like to consider? Make a point of finding out this information before you call them. It's far better to let them know you think they have such good potential that you have talked to your colleagues and found another position they might like to apply for. Even if they are not interested, they will remain positive about themselves and have positive memories of the whole process.

TAKE RISKS

If you know you have a similar vacancy coming up in another couple of months, consider taking the risk and employing one of the other good candidates as well. The turnover in nursing is so high that you could be foolish not to do so. Obviously you must get your finance advisor to work out all the costings and ensure you obtain your line manager's approval. It is usually a cost-effective way of dealing with things by the time you take into account the cost of further adverts and interviews.

ARRANGE A GOOD INDUCTION PROGRAMME

As soon as the candidate has confirmed their starting date, prepare their induction period together with your team. This is a crucial part of their employment. A good induction period makes the candidates feel welcome and reinforces their positive feelings about your ward. If you do not ensure this is done properly and then have problems later on with poor performance or incompetence, you could be found at fault because you failed to ensure an adequate induction period.

BEFORE THEY COMMENCE

You can start the induction before the candidate even starts the job by sending them any information that may be of interest together with a personal welcome letter from you. Include any forms that need signing to ensure they receive things in good time and save them unnecessary hassle, such as:

- car parking pass
- e-mail address and IT password
- ID badge and security pass
- uniform measurements.

Other items you might like to send them are:

- a copy of their 2-week initial induction programme
- a copy of their first roster with details of shift times
- a list of staff names in your team and any particular responsibilities, e.g. link nurse
- minutes from the last team meeting
- the name and details of their allocated mentor or preceptor.

TWO-WEEK SUPERNUMERARY PERIOD

It is advisable that the new recruit is supernumerary for the initial 2-week induction period (in addition to any formal organisational induction programme) making sure that they are not shown on the roster at all. If they are, there is the possibility that they may be used to cover in times of short staffing. You cannot afford to let this happen in those first few weeks. Their initial induction should include the following:

1. *A warm welcome on their first day*. Make sure you or a senior member of your staff are there to greet them and can spend some time going through things with them.
2. *An induction checklist*. Most organisations have an induction checklist to be completed. Encourage them to complete this over the first couple of months, not the first 2 weeks. Don't overload them with information.
3. *Mandatory training*. Try and fit all their annual mandatory study requirements within the 2-week supernumerary period. If you get the statutory sessions such as manual handling awareness, health and safety and basic life support out the way in the induction period, it will not impinge on the study time available for the rest of your team in that financial year.
4. *Clinical work*. Allocate time for working full or half shifts during the induction period. They need to get the practical experience working alongside members of your team. Don't allocate them patients to look after on their own without support. That is not induction, it is using them as a pair of hands.
5. *Attendance at meetings*. Take them along to any meetings you have. Let them observe the sisters' meeting and perhaps even meet the director of nursing if present. Give them an insight into your role, vision and values right at the beginning no matter how junior their grade. It would be good to do this with all new HCAs too.
6. *Attendance to individual needs*. Tailor each induction programme to each individual. If someone has just returned to work after some time out, their needs will be very different from someone who has transferred from another department within the same organisation.

It's a good idea to develop the induction programme with someone in your team of the same grade as the new recruit. They will be more understanding of the individual's needs.

ALLOCATE A PRECEPTOR OR CLINICAL SUPERVISOR

Allocate them a preceptor or clinical supervisor and ensure this person is rostered to work with them regularly. Most areas will have some sort of competency package for new members of staff to guide their skills development during the first few months. If you don't, you should. Following this, they should have their first appraisal at around 3–6 months to agree objectives and a personal development plan for the coming year. Don't neglect this part; it is very important.

CONTINUALLY EXPLORE ALL OTHER AVENUES TO GET STAFF

You can't afford to become complacent, even if you are 'up to establishment'. Always be on the lookout for new staff. If you create a warm and welcoming environment for anyone visiting your ward, you'll hopefully end up with a queue of people wanting to work there.

STUDENT NURSES

Word spreads quickly around student nurses about which wards are the best to work on, so make sure that all students allocated to your area are:

- warmly welcomed
- rostered to work with their mentor twice per week at the very least
- given lots of feedback about their progress
- invited to meetings.

If you do not receive students to your area because of your specialism, you will be losing out on a major source of future staff. Contact your local university and offer day- or week-long placements where students can shadow an experienced member of staff. Even spending a short time with you can make a huge impression.

BANK AND AGENCY STAFF

Some choose to work for the bank or agency on a permanent basis so that they can have more flexibility around their home life. However, they may change their minds and apply for a post on your ward if they see that they would have some choice over their shift patterns. In addition, make sure that your staff treat all bank and agency staff well by:

1. Greeting them each time with a warm welcome and full introductions.
2. Taking time to find out the person's name, qualifications and experience.
3. Taking time to show them around the ward and going through their patients' needs with them.
4. Continually checking on how they are doing throughout the shift.
5. Giving feedback on how they are doing (temporary staff rarely receive this unless they have done something wrong).
6. Giving thanks at the end of the shift for anything specific that they have achieved or done well, not just general thanks for turning up.

LIAISE CLOSELY WITH YOUR RECRUITMENT LEAD

Most health care organisations employ someone who deals solely with nursing recruitment. Their job is to make sure everything is being done to attract staff to your organisation. They will have knowledge of all current recruitment initiatives such as the cadet nursing programmes, return to practice courses and various job fairs. They will have a good idea of what vacancies are where, plus who is interviewing for what and when. If you keep in close contact with your recruitment lead they can let you know of promising candidates from elsewhere. They will also keep you informed about when the next 'batch' of students are due to finish and start looking for jobs.

The recruitment lead soon gets to know which wards are popular and which are not. They will deter promising students from the worst wards where it is known they will receive little support and attention. They do not want to put all that effort into recruiting staff who would leave within a few months due to unsatisfactory working conditions.

You cannot blame the national shortage of nurses for all your vacancies. Nurses are out there and to find them you have to put more time and effort into:

1. Making your ward one of the most popular wards to work on within your organisation.
2. Finding the right places and right times to recruit.

DON'T DISCRIMINATE

PART TIME DOES NOT MEAN PART SKILLED

Nursing remains a female-dominated profession and, as a result, there will always be a high percentage of part-time workers. Health care professionals usually start off their careers working full time, but many will reduce to part time at some time during their careers in order to balance family and work commitments. This does not mean that they should be demoted or passed over for promotion. Don't assume that because a person does not want to work full time they are not as highly committed and motivated as those who do. If you do, you are being discriminatory

In addition to this, some part-time workers will not apply for promotion because they have the impression that a higher grade means working more hours. Try not to condone this culture; a higher grade means that higher skills are needed, not a higher number of hours.

If you do need to cover a certain number of shifts with a certain level of skill then consider employing two people to share one job. Two people sharing one job will give you far more than one person in terms of experience. (You have to be careful that they are truly job sharing, i.e. not working the same shifts.) The key to this working successfully is to ensure they jointly take responsibility for the one role. In other words, they can't blame the other for not getting things done.

OVERSEAS NURSES ARE NOT ALL THE SAME

You may be familiar with the following expressions from nurses within organisations who have recruited from another country:

● 'They are all so hard working.'
● 'They don't understand that nursing is different here.'
● 'Where they come from, they do what the doctors tell them to.'
● 'They are quick to learn our ways.'
● 'They demand so much of our time.'

We would not dream of stereotyping all UK nurses in such a manner, because we accept that they are all individuals. Yet people will often take the attitude that nurses who train in another country are all the same. Be careful not to condone this attitude. Accept that all these nurses are individuals, with their own unique blend of strengths and weaknesses. Work on their strengths as you would any other new member of staff.

Overseas recruitment is a fantastic opportunity to bring in new ideas and different experiences to your team. It may be a hassle to ensure they have the appropriate competences and skills for the role but no more than any other staff nurse you recruit to your team. If you have a new recruit who is struggling in the role, look to improving your own systems of support and methods of staff development before blaming the individual nurse. If you undervalue individuals in any way, you will undermine their confidence and self-esteem. It will not help them work well. If you value each individual for the unique qualities that they bring to the team, they will feel good about themselves and consequently be motivated to work well.

SUCCESSION PLAN

IS YOUR STAFFING ESTABLISHMENT CONDUCIVE TO GOOD SUCCESSION PLANNING?

Think carefully about the mix of grades within your staffing establishment. If you only have one deputy, for example, you could be limiting promotion prospects for your staff. Having two deputy managers rather than one may be more helpful in terms of succession planning. If you have ten staff nurses and only one deputy, you may be putting yourself at risk of losing good staff who will look elsewhere to get in the next grade. It also reflects poorly on you if one of your senior staff leaves and you have nobody in your team who is ready to replace them. If this does happen, review and improve on what you are doing to develop the skills of your team.

STAFF NURSE LEVEL (BAND 5)

Since the advent of pay bands, the perpetual headache of having two grades of staff nurse has finally been removed. It became quite ridiculous having to interview D grades for E grade jobs, which only served to hinder rather than help staff retention. Things are a lot easier now that all staff nurses are in band 5. However, having one staff nurse grade does not mean you can forgo any thoughts of succession planning. You still need to ensure they are competent enough to get through that gateway halfway through the pay band. You also need some system in place so they have the opportunity to get to deputy manager/ward sister standard (band 6) over a certain time span.

Good succession planning means that when senior people leave you will have at least one person who is up to the standard of taking on that role. Make sure you have a system in place so that each staff nurse who joins your team has a detailed personal development plan linked to the knowledge and skills framework (KSF). This should give them every opportunity to be able to get through the mid-point gateway. Do the same for your senior staff nurses to get to the level where they can apply for the next pay band.

Your recruitment plan for registered nurses should continually aim for the newly qualified or junior staff nurse level; however, don't always promote internally. It is good to regularly employ nurses higher up the pay band scale from external sources.

They will bring valuable experience, new ideas and, more importantly, they will challenge your ways of working.

DEPUTY MANAGER/SISTER/CHARGE NURSE LEVEL (BAND 6)

Be on constant lookout for your next deputy(s). If any of your staff nurses have particularly good management and organisational skills, you will want to develop those skills and get them ready for when your current deputy(s) decides to leave. Don't wait until people resign before looking around to replace them. Be proactive and ensure you have staff ready to take on the post should the opportunity arise.

HEALTH CARE ASSISTANTS

You should also provide a system of career progression within your staffing establishment for HCAs. They should be able to access diploma level 2, then level 3 and even level 4. They may not wish to progress any further than their current level but the opportunity to do so should always be there. Some may prefer to specialise into areas such as taking on a link role or diversifying into taking on some ward administrative duties. As with the registered nurses, when a senior HCA leaves, you should have at least one other HCA ready to take their place.

FULLY INVOLVE YOUR TEAM IN ALL ASPECTS OF RECRUITMENT

People sometimes get the words 'inform' and 'involve' confused. Involving your team in the recruitment process entails more than just ensuring they are fully informed at each stage of the process. Keeping them fully informed is better than nothing but it will be far more beneficial to go one step further and actually involve them all in the process.

As soon as any team member resigns, meet your team to review the role and discuss whether it should remain the same or whether a different role would further enhance the team. Involve them in redesigning the job description if that is needed.

When you are ready to write the advert, get your team together to discuss and agree how to word the advert to make it more attractive to potential candidates. If you do not have time to meet with all your team, use other means of communication. Add it to the agenda of your regular team meetings rather than set up a special meeting.

DEVELOP THEIR INTERVIEWING SKILLS EARLY ON

Include at least one of your team in the interviewing process. Guidelines usually recommend that at least one of the interviewers should be a higher grade than the candidate. There is no reason why you cannot include someone from your team who is the same or even a lower grade than that of the candidate; they have to start somewhere. Don't wait until staff nurses become a band 6 before inviting them to sit in on interviews. The experience is extremely valuable. If they are only observing, give them one of the questions to ask. Everyone remembers their first interview when they had to ask questions and were too nervous to listen to the candidate's reply. It's something that should be done at an early stage in people's careers and not left until they are deputy or ward manager level (as is so often the case).

Take time after the interviews not only to discuss and agree the successful candidate but also to discuss the process. If you have a team member with you who is new to the process, ask what they have learned. Discuss the process with the whole panel. Was there anything you felt you could have done better?

GET THE TEAM INVOLVED WITH THE NEW STAFF MEMBER EARLY ON

Once you have offered the post, let your team know who the new team member is and a bit about their background, then immediately appoint someone to take the lead in planning their induction. Make sure your culture of involving all the team also applies in turn to team members. In other words, encourage the person planning the induction to ask the rest of the team for their ideas on what should be included.

If you can, get someone of the same grade as the new team member to sort out the induction programme. They will understand the new person's needs better than anyone else. That includes HCAs; you do not need to be a registered nurse to be able to organise an induction programme for an HCA.

The key to having robust recruitment and retention is to ensure you show that you value the input from all your team members. It's the fundamental difference between leading your team and managing your team. Lead them well during the process and you will have a far stronger and healthier team than if you simply administer the recruitment process yourself.

ACTION POINTS

- Each time a member of your staff leaves, review the post and job description with the 'leaver' and the rest of your team.
- Involve your team in writing job adverts and customising the application packages for your ward.
- Include the interview date on all adverts and shortlist within 5 days of the closing date.
- Include your team in the whole process. Ensure at least one team member is included in the interview process and ensure all prospective candidates are given a warm welcome by your team when visiting the ward.
- Make sure all new team members receive a 2-week supernumerary induction programme devised by your staff and including mandatory updates.
- Network widely to ensure that you and your team are continually aware of new recruitment opportunities.
- Review your staffing establishment and systems of developing your staff to ensure they have every opportunity to develop the skills for the next post and are ready within 2–3 years of commencement in their current role.
- If you do not already do so, start involving your team in the whole process of recruitment rather than just keeping them informed.

Reference

Health and Safety Executive, 2011. Management standards for work related stress – demands. Online. Available: http://www.hse.gov.uk/stress/standards/demands.htm Feb 2012.

CHAPTER 9

BE POLITICALLY AWARE

Being politically aware means knowing how your organisation ticks, who's who and how to use this knowledge to get things done. Without this knowledge, you can become cocooned in your own small environment. You may be taken advantage of because of your ignorance. You also run the risk of missing out on opportunities to improve your working environment, your staff and patient care. To be a good manager, it is essential that you know:

- how your own organisation and other health care organisations operate
- the health strategy and policy at a national and local level and how to take account of them when planning your goals with your team
- who the key people are who can make things happen (both internally and external to your organisation) and how to get hold of them.

A good manager should learn how to network and build strong alliances in order to become more powerful and effective in the role.

UNDERSTAND HOW HEALTH CARE IS MANAGED NATIONALLY

The general public thinks of the NHS across the United Kingdom (which is made up of England, Wales, Scotland and Northern Ireland) as one system, but this is not quite true. The common thread is they are all funded through the taxation system, something which differentiates the UK health system from that of almost all other countries, as well as adhering to the principle of offering free care to all. Each of the four countries has important differences in the way it spends its money in pursuing the goal of free health care for all. To complicate things further, new 'top-down' initiatives emanate from Whitehall with increasing frequency, and so major reorganisations of the NHS in England are now a matter of course, with the inevitable modifications to this in Scotland, Wales and Northern Ireland.

If you want to understand and perhaps even to challenge enforced changes within your workplace, knowing what the current key strategies and policies of your part of the NHS are, from where they originate and how they affect your day-to-day practice is essential.

THE NHS IN ENGLAND

The Department of Health sets the national standards and shapes the direction of the NHS in England. It sets out the priorities for the NHS each year in a document entitled *The NHS Operating Framework*. The work of the Department of Health is supported by various bodies known as Arm's Length Bodies (or 'quasi non-governmental organisations' colloquially known as 'quangos'). These include the Care Quality Commission (CQC), Monitor and the National Institute for Health and Clinical Excellence (NICE).

GPs are deemed to be at the pivot of the NHS in England. The commissioning groups led by the GPs receive around 80% of the NHS budget, which they then spend on purchasing services from NHS trusts and other providers. In theory, since GPs should commission high-quality providers rather than those who provide poor-quality service, standards should rise over time. Indeed, the commissioning groups can even withhold a percentage of payments if the agreed quality standards are not met. These include standards for which you are responsible such as the number of patient falls, incidents or complaints, or even the levels of staffing.

In addition, the Department of Health employs a chief nursing officer (CNO) for England, who is the most senior nurse advisor to the government. Accessing the Department of Health Web site (www.dh.gov.uk) regularly is a wise move for all nurse managers. It gives updated information about relevant issues in the NHS which have an impact on all nurses and midwives. It also enables you to access link Web sites to obtain further information about issues that will affect your work.

THE NHS IN WALES, SCOTLAND AND NORTHERN IRELAND

Wales, Scotland and Northern Ireland have not adopted the system of commissioning between purchasers (GPs) and providers (hospitals), i.e. the 'internal market'. Instead, each country has a system of regional health bodies which plan and commission all hospital, GP and other health care services for their local populations. In Wales and Scotland they are called health or NHS boards; in Northern Ireland they are called health and social care trusts. Each country has its own Department of Health responsible for policy direction, and a body similar to the CQC for setting national clinical standards, ensuring they are put into practice and monitoring performance. Although the health systems are managed separately, there is some overlap; for example, the NICE guidelines currently apply to both Wales and England.

Each country in the UK also has its own CNO as their most senior nurse advisor. For further information, see:

- NHS Wales: www.wales.nhs.uk
- NHS Scotland: www.show.scot.nhs.uk
- NHS Northern Ireland: www.n-i.nhs.uk.

PRIVATE HEALTH CARE

At the time of writing this book there are various private companies in the UK providing acute care, the biggest being BMI Healthcare which has over 70 hospitals, closely followed by Spire Healthcare with 37 hospitals, Nuffield Health with 32 hospitals, and Ramsay Health Care UK with 22 hospitals across the UK. There are many other smaller companies. Private hospitals base their standards along the relevant NHS regulations and guidelines. In England, they have to register with the CQC and thus meet the same care quality standards as the NHS.

BE AWARE OF THE WIDER ORGANISATION

This is basic information about how health care is run in the UK. If you did not know much of it before, do rest assured that you are not alone. Nurses are often so focused on managing their day-to-day pressures that being aware of the wider organisation has never been a priority. However, once you become a nurse manager, you will find it helpful to become more aware of the 'bigger picture'. Don't fall into the trap of thinking that 'what happens out there does not concern me' or 'I haven't got time for that'. If you do not know how the system works, you cannot influence it.

Make it a personal goal from now on to keep yourself abreast of the ongoing changes both nationally and within your own organisation. All this information is now freely available on the relevant NHS Web sites (national or local). Because it is for the general public, it is easy and quick to read as most of the jargon tends to be removed.

KNOW YOUR BOARD OF DIRECTORS AND THEIR PRIORITIES

In England, all NHS trusts have a board of directors, who are collectively accountable for the organisation. Every trust board is required to have a chairman and a mix of executive and non-executive directors.

Generally, the board comprises the following members:

- Chairman × 1,
- Chief executive × 1,
- Executive directors × 5 (or more),
- Non-executive directors × 5 (or more),

Non-executive directors

The chairman is a non-executive role. The chairman and non-executive directors are generally non-clinical people whose role is to give an independent voice, provide a level of scrutiny and make sure that the trust board is working in the interests of the local community. Some might have business or financial skills whereas others may have experience as a carer or even as a patient. The chairman and non-executive directors are not responsible for the operational management of the organisation. The idea is that they bring an independent and enquiring perspective to help the board to ensure a high-quality service. They are expected to draw from their experiences to make sure that the patients' interests are paramount.

Both the chairman and non-executive directors are employed part-time on 4-year contracts. The chairman usually works 3 days per week and the non-executive directors work 2–5 days per month.

The chairman

The chairman's role is to lead the trust board and ensure it fulfils all its responsibilities. The role entails chairing all the board meetings and ensuring the smooth running of the board by supporting, constructively challenging and setting the appropriate tone for the way the board works. The chairman's other main role is to communicate effectively both internally and externally to gain the views and commitment from the staff and the local community. This is why you'll often see the chairman walking around the organisation with staff and attending various community and organisational events.

The chairman appoints the chief executive who then appoints the executive directors.

Executive directors

Of the five executive director members, the following are a statutory requirement:

- Chief executive.
- Director of finance.
- Medical director.
- Director of nursing and midwifery.

The fifth executive director and any further appointments are at the discretion of the trust. Some appoint an executive director for human resources. Others may decide on having an executive director for operations or planning. In addition to the five executive directors, there may be a small number of further directors who are not in an executive role. This means that they attend board meetings but do not have voting rights.

Executive directors are responsible for a particular function within the organisation such as nursing or finance, but as board members they are required to contribute to other trust-wide issues and policy outside their particular brief. All directors of the board have a corporate responsibility for:

- setting the strategic direction
- ensuring effective financial planning and control
- promoting quality and clinical governance
- agreeing annual business plans.

The chief executive

The chief executive has personal responsibility for the overall operational management of the organisation and reports to the chairman. The chief executive is accountable for the trust's performance both in terms of meeting statutory requirements such as financial stability and health and safety legislation, and also quality targets.

GETTING TO KNOW YOUR BOARD OF DIRECTORS

The board of directors is a very powerful body, so it makes sense to build alliances and networks with some of the key players on the board so you can benefit. The director of nursing is the nurse with the greatest authority within the organisation, yet it has been found that nearly 40% of nurses do not even know who their nursing director is (Royal College of Nursing 2010). The board usually holds a meeting in public every month. Anyone can attend to listen and ask questions. Going along to these board meetings is an easy way of getting to know and understand what is going on. Take staff along for the experience and to help develop their political awareness.

Many chief executives also hold regular 'open forums'. They book a couple of hours in their diaries where they will be available at a certain venue for anyone to come along and ask questions. These are not only information-giving meetings; they are there for the staff to raise and discuss any issues or concerns.

Another easy way of finding out what your trust board's priorities and plans are is via the intranet or in the annual business plan. This plan is open to the public and therefore written in an easily readable style. You need to know what your board's priorities are. If the priorities of your ward or department are different from those of the trust board, you will not get very far with them.

For those working in private health care, the system is less complex, but it is necessary that you make yourself aware of what your company's priorities are, if you have not already done so.

CHOOSE YOUR MEETINGS CAREFULLY

Select your meetings carefully; this is not only for time management reasons. There are certain meetings that you should attend and contribute to, to ensure you are part of the organisation's important network and remain up-to-date with what is going on. As a general rule, if the person chairing the meeting is not particularly influential within your organisation and does not have the authority to make decisions, then think twice before going; your time could be better spent.

BOARD MEETINGS

The monthly meetings of the trust board are extremely useful. It is worth putting the dates in your diary to remind you to organise yourself or one of your team to attend that day. Add it to the top of the roster to remind your team about it. It will also make them realise the importance of the role of the board (and perhaps even to keep them aware that there is one!).

Consider adding an attendance at a trust board meeting to your staff induction programme. It will stimulate their thinking about the wider organisation. In addition, the directors will probably note the continual attendance of members of your team. It can do you no harm to be seen as a forward-thinking manager within the organisation.

SISTERS' MEETINGS

Many nursing directors hold regular sisters' meetings in order to:

- find out what is going on at ward level
- gain your views and opinions (which will influence decision making at board level)
- discuss any issues that are currently affecting your practice
- keep you informed about any changes in policies or guidance
- get you involved in specific projects for improving patient care.

Add the dates of sisters' meetings to your roster too. They are very important and often your only access to the director of nursing. You will not be able to attend every time, so always make sure that at least two of your senior staff members are familiar with the meeting structure. They will then be able to attend in your absence with confidence.

DIRECTORATE MEETINGS

Most NHS organisations are divided into directorates, divisions or business units. Meetings at this level are just as important for you to attend. If you do not, decisions will be made without your input but may affect your work. Prepare for these meetings; look at the agenda beforehand. Think about anything you need to know or ask about. Do not go to meetings just with the intention of getting information. That is a waste of your time. It will be quicker to read the minutes. Go to meetings prepared in order to contribute and influence decisions.

SENDING STAFF TO MEETINGS ON YOUR BEHALF

Try not to send any members of staff to meetings without prior experience. The main reason for sending a substitute to a meeting is to contribute to the decision-making processes. Putting a member of staff in a room full of senior colleagues for the first time and expecting them to speak confidently on your behalf is expecting too much. It could be quite a damaging experience. Whenever you can, take a member of your staff along with you to meetings to gain the appropriate experience. Once they are familiar with the process, you will be able to send them along as your representative when you cannot attend in person.

Try and ensure you are always represented at every board, directorate and sisters' meeting. Never be concerned about missing out on important information. You will get all the information you need from the minutes. The main reason for attending meetings is to contribute, on behalf of your staff, to future changes and development within your organisation. It is important that you are part of the nursing agenda in your trust. Staff on induction would also benefit by coming along with you to observe.

IMPROMPTU MEETINGS

Prepare for impromptu meetings with influential people. Chairmen are often found wandering around hospitals meeting people to get a feel for what is going on. That's their job. Don't just say hello and generally pass the time of day. Prepare in advance something that you would want to say or ask, in the event that you may pass them one day in the corridor. You may even have a politician or the media visit your trust. These visits are often booked with very little notice. It is a good idea to always have at least one question in your mind should such a situation arise, to avoid it becoming a wasted opportunity.

NETWORK – GET TO KNOW THE RIGHT PEOPLE

The right people to know are not necessarily the most senior people. Often they are the secretaries or teams who work for senior people. Medical secretaries, for example, have a wealth of information about what is going on. The personal assistant who works for the chief executive or director of nursing is also a very useful person to know. They know how their boss thinks and are usually full of very helpful advice.

Always smile and say hello when you walk in through your hospital reception. Stop every now and then to pass the time of day. Do the same with the porters, the people who serve you in the canteen and the person who mops the corridor outside your ward each day. The more people you know, the more you will get to know about what is happening in your organisation.

OTHER WARD MANAGERS

You should also cultivate a good friendship with your peers. Working in isolation from the managers of other wards and departments will weaken your influence in the organisation. Get together with the others as a group and you will strengthen your position and voice. Try and ensure you support and help each other in times of pressure.

SENIOR MANAGERS AND DIRECTORS

Get to know the senior managers. Don't shy away from them. One way to do this is to hang back after meetings where senior managers are involved. Usually after such a meeting, the clinical staff dash back to their familiar clinical environment, but it is worth staying behind for a short while. Tidy up the coffee cups or put the chairs back in order to stop you feeling awkward. You may find you are drawn into a conversation with a senior manager asking you for your opinion about something from a clinical perspective. The more you do this, the more you will become confident in speaking with them.

BE ALERT TO OPPORTUNITIES

Take your time to develop your alliances. It will not happen overnight. Just be alert to opportunities for getting to know the right people. They will not come to you; you have to go out and find them. Having the appropriate networks can mean the difference between success or failure in your role.

BUILDING UP YOUR NETWORKS

Networking is about building a two-way alliance. You should be prepared to give more than you receive. Tips for increasing your networks include:

- *Helping others out*. Offer to send some information about something you have talked about and ensure you follow it up. Nobody forgets a simple, friendly gesture like this. Make sure you add your contact details on your cover note.
- *Saying thank you*. If you hear an interesting speaker at a meeting or teaching session, go up afterwards and thank the speaker. People rarely do this but speakers do appreciate some feedback. This may or may not spark up a short conversation, which you could follow up afterwards. Whatever the outcome, they will remember you.

Remember that the junior staff you come across such as medical and nursing students may well get to be in more senior and influential positions than you one day. Try to ensure that they always remember you in a positive light.

BE DIPLOMATIC

GUARD YOUR OPINIONS

Know when to keep your opinions to yourself. Don't express your point of view unless you have been requested to do so. People who offer opinions without being asked can be irritating. They tend to do so because:

- they have an audience
- they want to make people think they are clever
- they want to get attention
- they think it will make a difference.

Learn when to say something and when to keep quiet. Opinions don't usually make a difference unless they have been asked for. When you are asked for your thoughts or judgements, try to avoid using phrases such as 'in my opinion'. It would be better to present your opinion as a solution. For example:

Question: 'What do you think about the changes in the admission procedure?'
Answer 1: 'Well, in my opinion, the paperwork takes too long to complete.'
Answer 2: 'The paperwork could certainly be reviewed. It takes too long to complete.'

The second answer sounds like a well-considered answer. The person is confident and appears to know what they are talking about. Opinions are more likely to be accepted if presented as a fact rather than as an opinion, if they are presented in a confident and adept manner.

TRY NOT TO BE TOO CRITICAL

If you have problems with a colleague or a senior manager, don't criticise them personally. If you think a senior manager is lazy or incompetent, never say so. Getting personal is not professional. On the other hand, you cannot ignore a senior manager's behaviour if it is affecting others. You just need to be diplomatic about it. Focus on the behaviour, not the person. You could say, for example, that perhaps they need to increase their motivation or update their clinical skills.

DON'T TAKE SIDES

Don't take sides in times of conflict between others. As soon as you do this, you become part of the dispute. Stay objective, remain calm and don't be drawn in. You will come across as more confident and self-assured. Calming down situations of conflict also gets you noticed in a positive light. In the same way, getting into heated arguments is totally unprofessional. You will be seen in a negative way, no matter how right you are.

CONTROL YOUR TEMPER

If a major decision has been made without your consultation, do not create an argument and never become aggressive. Always think very carefully before you act. These are times when a mentor or clinical supervisor may help you find an alternative way of dealing with the situation.

Usually there is nothing you can do other than accept a bad decision, but take action to ensure something similar never happens again. Always learn from your experiences. It is usually best to let the individual(s) know how you feel about the decision but then leave it at that. Don't let these things fester. After all, it is only a job!

TALK OF 'WE' RATHER THAN 'I'

Having the right attitude makes all the difference. You may find some of your colleagues develop a 'them and us' attitude. They like to side with their staff and moan about 'the management'. Try not to become one of them; your staff will not respect you, nor will the management. Besides, you are now part of the management. Even if you do not agree with some managerial decisions, try to keep your adverse feelings away from your staff. Just stick to the facts when explaining the situation to your team. If you talk of 'we' rather than 'I', you automatically assume a position of greater authority when talking to others.

THINK AS A MANAGER

When problems occur, it is easy to see things from your own point of view, but it is the manager's role to regard things from the team and organisational perspective.

Don't waste time thinking:

- 'Will this mean I will have to work more weekends?'
- 'What do I get if I put us forward to be part of the pilot project?'
- 'Will this make me look good?'

Consider things from a managerial point of view:

- 'How can I ensure adequate senior cover at weekends?'
- 'Will this pilot project improve patient care?'
- 'How will this benefit the staff?'

REPRESENT YOUR ORGANISATION

There are some ward managers who have not grasped the concept of being part of an organisation. This becomes apparent when something goes wrong. Phrases such as, 'It's not our fault. It was the admissions department who cancelled your appointment, not us' or, 'Sorry, there are no pillows, the linen service here is terrible' may reflect the true facts of a situation but this is not the stance a manager should take.

Always remember that you are representing your organisation as one of its managers. If patients complain about services that have nothing to do with your department, empathise and reassure them that you will relay their concerns to the appropriate people to ensure that services will improve. Don't be defensive.

VOICING YOUR DISAGREEMENTS

If you do disagree with something, be careful how you do it. You may wish to say, for example, 'If we are going to open up four more beds, we need to consider how it will affect the team' instead of, 'I think you're mad to even suggest it'. There will always be disagreements with others within your organisation; just be careful about how you deal with them.

WORK WITH YOUR DIRECTOR OF NURSING

The director of nursing is an executive director. This is a very powerful position. They have far greater authority than your line manager and even your general manager. The director of nursing is the professional lead for nurses throughout the organisation. They work closely with the chief executive and other board directors in making decisions about what happens in the organisation overall.

The majority of nursing directors do not directly manage the nursing workforce, so some nurses get the impression that their role is not important; they could not be more wrong. You should make it your goal to build a strong alliance with your director of nursing.

THE PROFESSIONAL DEVELOPMENT TEAM

The director of nursing is responsible for the professional development of the nursing workforce and will usually have a small team of senior nurses to assist them in this role. This includes one or more deputy directors and various practice development nurses. It is a wise move to develop close working relationships with the deputy director(s) and practice development team. Their role is to help you develop practice, so you should make maximum use of this resource. Much of their work is currently dictated by national and local policy so close liaison will help keep you abreast of new policies and procedures.

SHADOWING

Try and arrange to spend a day shadowing your nursing director if you can, to give you an insight into the role and responsibilities. If you feel too awkward approaching them out of the blue, introduce the idea via an e-mail. Make it short and succinct. Point out that you would like to learn more about their role and to pick up tips about how you can manage your ward more effectively. Many directors welcome this approach as it also gives them a chance to get to know more about what is happening at a clinical level in your area. They will let you know what dates they have available which will be appropriate for your learning.

MENTORING

Following the shadowing experience, it may be an idea to follow it up with a request for mentoring for the next 6 months. Having a director of nursing as a mentor for a while would be an invaluable experience. You will benefit from lots of hints and tips to help you in your current role. You may have the added benefit of increasing your networks as they introduce you to other senior members in your organisation. The greater your network, the more influential you will become.

Your nursing director will also get to know you. They will see that you run a good ward, that you are forward thinking and that you have leadership potential. When opportunities arise, they may think of you first of all as the person who may benefit. They may have access to some funding, for example, to assist with a project. If you had mentioned that it is something you are currently working on, you may find that you are nominated for the funding. Keeping your director informed of your work can bring all sorts of benefits.

Being closely associated with your director of nursing will give you the opportunity to influence the wider agenda and contribute to any major decisions affecting your organisation. But it will not just happen; you have to make it happen.

GET RECOGNITION FOR YOUR WORK

If you don't get to know the right people, your work and that of your team will have less chance of being recognised and appreciated. Celebrate your successes and let the rest of the organisation know how good your team are.

HOSPITAL NEWSLETTER/INTRANET

Write something regularly for your hospital newsletter. You do not have to be an accomplished journalist. The communications team are there to help you. Try not to just use the newsletter as a way of keeping people up-to-date with matters such as 'Staff nurse Sam Jones just had a baby' or 'Sister Smith has been promoted'. Talk about any innovations or changes that have made an improvement to patient care. Put forward ideas that other wards may benefit from. It could be something like a successful change in your handover system or how a new system of restricted visiting times helped your patients get a much-needed rest.

One of the board directors usually has to read through and approve the newsletter before it is finally distributed. Your team's contributions will not go unnoticed.

CONFERENCES AND STUDY DAYS

Encourage your staff to speak about their successes at local workshops and conferences. You can find out about these through your organisation's practice development team. Keep them informed and involved in all new initiatives on your ward. They will hopefully tell others of your good work and help promote it to others too.

COMPARE YOUR WARD WITH OTHERS

There is nothing more soul-destroying than to read an article or see people being praised for implementing a new way of working that you've been doing for years. The problem is being able to recognise the things you do that are better than other areas. One of the best ways of doing this is to spend time working with a member of staff who has recently joined you from another area. Having a student nurse work closely with you for a day is a great way of finding out what people do on other wards and to point out what things you do well on your ward.

The benchmarking process is another good way of finding out what you do well in comparison with other areas. Promoting the work of your team is not a selfish thing to do. It is recognising their hard work and rewarding them for a job well done.

CHOOSE YOUR MENTOR AND MENTEES WITH CARE

THE MENTOR ROLE

When you become a manager, it is wise to have a mentor who is a lot more senior than yourself. The role of a mentor is to provide advice, guidance, information and contacts to help you in your work (for a definition of mentoring for managers, see p. 180). A good mentor can be invaluable because:

- they have far more experience than you
- they have often 'been there and done it' before
- they will help you benefit from the knowledge they have in their current position
- they can introduce you to their wider networks.

Aim high

Try not to settle for someone who is just one or two grades above you; aim higher. The more senior your mentor is within your organisation, the more they can help you become influential in your role. A member of the board is ideal. A non-executive director in particular can give you the benefits of their skills from outside the NHS. They are usually keen to take on the mentor role because they want to understand your role better. Having a mentee at clinical level gives them a valuable insight into the complexities of running a ward.

Your mentor may be able to explain how to get certain things done. If you feel you need extra staff for your unit and are getting nowhere, having a finance manager as your mentor can be extremely advantageous. Don't expect them to do things for you; it's not that easy. However, you can get them to explain the system clearly to you and point out where you are going wrong.

Don't choose a mentor who has little or no influence in your organisation. It will be a waste of time. If they have no influence, how can they help you to gain those skills? How will they help increase your networks? Managers within the NHS who are not politically aware do not make good mentors.

Change your mentor as necessary

You don't have to keep the same mentor all the time. Set a limited time span such as 6–8 months to start with. By this time you will have got to know them well and can choose to either stay with them or move on.

CHOOSING YOUR MENTEES

It is advisable not to have more than a maximum of three people to mentor. Your time is precious. Don't waste your time on people who are only looking for your help to improve their career prospects. Watch for staff who have good potential. You'll know them when you see them. They are usually committed, hard working and produce high standards of work. Sometimes they don't know they are good. Their work may go unnoticed. Only you are experienced enough to know that with a bit of extra guidance and support, this person could go a long way and really make a difference.

Being a mentor to someone with potential can be a very rewarding experience through watching them become more confident in themselves with your guidance and support. They may well become more senior than you one day. It can give a huge sense of satisfaction knowing that you were part of the process. And what's more, they'll never forget you.

Steer clear of your own junior team members

Try not to mentor a junior member of your own team unless it is your deputy. It may cause resentment among the rest of the team. If you do have someone in your team that you feel would flourish with good mentoring, ask one of your colleagues (fellow ward managers) to become their mentor.

Mentoring new ward managers

It's a good idea to get together with your peers and set up a system whereby the more experienced ward managers mentor the newer and less experienced ones. No ward manager should start their new role without being assigned a more experienced manager to mentor them. Show them the ropes. Introduce them to the essential people and systems they need to know to get things done. Don't let them struggle like you probably did. A good internal mentoring system will build a stronger team of ward managers within your organisation.

PLAN AHEAD FOR YOUR OWN NEEDS

Don't neglect your own needs. Being politically aware can also help you with where you want to go. Have you thought about where are you heading? You may wish to go into management, education or a more senior specialist clinical role (e.g. nurse consultant). Even if you want to stay where you are until retirement, it is still wise to plan ahead to ensure you get the best out of your job.

IDENTIFY YOUR SPECIFIC INTERESTS

If your ultimate aim is to become a nurse consultant, start specialising in your subject now. Become a member of the appropriate specialist association and ask the appropriate clinical nurse specialist or medical consultant to become your mentor.

If your aim is to go into senior management or teaching, you would benefit by developing your skills in a particular area. Make sure that your name is linked with the specialist interest throughout the organisation. You could join the appropriate project group or perhaps even write an article for one of the mainstream nursing journals. Get yourself recognised. Don't leave it to chance. That ideal job won't just fall in your lap; you have to make it happen.

It is easy to allow your own needs to get overlooked when your time is taken up with meeting the needs of your patients and staff. Boosting your individual status is something nurses find hard to do. You have to make your mark so you stand out and your potential is noticed. Having a specific area of interest will enable you to do this. Although your job requires you to have a general knowledge of all issues, becoming an expert in one or two specific areas can help your future career prospects.

KEEP A FILE FOR YOUR CV

It is doubtful if anyone has the time or inclination to keep their CV up-to-date at all times, but it is helpful to keep a file (electronic or paper) and each time you attend a course, workshop or study session, add any relevant papers, certificates or reflective notes. You'll find it easier when you come to writing your application, to have everything together in one place rather than having to search through papers and e-mails trying to remember what you did.

WRITING YOUR CV

The basic outline of a CV (see Appendix 9.1 for a sample CV) should contain the following:

● Your name.
● Your address.
● Your contact details.
● A summary of your current role.

Write a brief couple of paragraphs outlining your current role. This is one of the most important parts of your CV. Don't use the job description. Everyone knows the responsibilities of a ward manager. Promote what is special about you.

A summary of your educational achievements

List these in date order starting with the most recent courses. You don't need to include your school education; you are too senior for that to matter now. Your registered nurse qualification/degree should be the last one on the list.

A summary of your work experience

List your roles and the organisations where you have worked since registering as a nurse. Put these in date order starting with the most recent experience. Don't repeat your current role here. You have already outlined this at the beginning of the document. Write in any key achievements. Don't list what your responsibilities were as staff nurse. They are well known. You need to convince your new employer that you are a person who achieves things, rather than just does what is listed in the job description.

References

Two references are required, one from your current employer and one from your previous employer. If you have been in your current post for many years, you could use someone else like a link lecturer or course tutor. (Remember always to ask your referees first. Never just assume that they will provide one. It is inconsiderate to put down someone's name as a reference without asking.)

TAILOR YOUR CV/APPLICATION FORM TO THE JOB

Each CV or application form should be tailored to the job you are applying for. Don't be tempted to include everything. No matter how senior or experienced you are, your CV should never be more than two pages long. Your potential employers need to see that you have the relevant skills for the job. They do not want to wade through everything you have done and have to try to decipher for themselves which bits are relevant.

ACTION POINTS

- Access the appropriate Web sites each month to keep yourself up-to-date with what's going on nationally.
- Find out the membership of your organisation's board and what their priorities are.
- Aim to attend or send a representative to all the board meetings, sisters' meetings and local directorate/divisional meetings.
- Aim to add at least one new contact to your network every few months.
- Concentrate on presenting facts when asked your opinion and never criticise others.
- Never use the phrase 'the management'.
- Make a date to shadow your director of nursing.
- Write a short article for your hospital's newsletter about a recent achievement in your ward or department.
- Get yourself a senior mentor.
- Consider whether your current mentees are relevant.
- If you have not already done so, start a file (electronic or paper) for your CV/next application form.

Reference

Royal College of Nursing, 2010. New foundations: the future of NHS trust providers: Policy briefing 05/2010. Online. Available: http://www.rcn.org.uk/__data/assets/pdf_file/0006/314619/05.10_New_Foundations_the_future_of_NHS_Trust_Providers_Report.pdf Feb 2012.

SAMPLE CV

Jane Smith
21 St James Street, Newbury, Gloucestershire GN23 4FN
Tel: 08900 400300
E-mail: *jane.smith@internet.com*

Current role: Ward Manager, Flower Ward, Tree NHS Trust from 2008 to present

I manage a 28-bed medical ward, using a primary nursing model, which I successfully implemented 4 years ago. I manage a team of 35 staff with a budget of £1.2m. I use a bottom-up leadership approach in all aspects of my work by ensuring that I involve my team in all decisions and encouraging them to consistently challenge the status quo. I have a particular interest in the care of patients admitted with endocrine disorders and have developed a special interest group together with the diabetes specialist nurse on the care of patients with newly diagnosed diabetes.

Educational achievements

Dec 2012 MSc in Health Service Management, University of London.
Jan 2006 BSc Professional Nursing Studies, University of London.
Feb 2002 RN, PgDip (PIN 123456 Exp 05/10), University of Surrey.

Career history

2006–2008 Senior Staff Nurse (band 6), Stroke Unit, Another Trust, London.
Key achievements: Successful implementation of team nursing; instrumental in reducing staff vacancies from 50% on commencement of role to no vacancies within 1 year.
2004–2006 Staff Nurse (band 5), 26-bed Medical/Endocrine Ward, Another Trust, Surrey.
Key achievements: Development of an in-house 1-year training programme to develop the skills of newly qualified nurses in caring for medical patients.
2002–2004 Staff Nurse (band 5), 28-bed Medical/Respiratory Ward, Another Trust, Surrey.

References

Current employer
Mrs A Smith
Medical Unit
Tree NHS Trust
08900 000000
jdeq@internet.com

Senior Lecturer
Mr B Jones
Faculty of Health and Social Care
University of London
08900 333333
jq@university.com

CHAPTER 10

LOOK AFTER YOURSELF

Taking on the role of a manager gives you greater power and authority. However, this power and authority comes at a price: your staff will have greater expectations. They will require you to:

- support them through difficult times
- take over in situations when they don't know what to do
- provide the appropriate resources and environment to enable them to do their job properly
- know everything
- be confident
- always make the right decisions
- never be off sick
- never have any problems of your own
- never make mistakes.

When you were a staff nurse, you were safe in the knowledge that there was someone more knowledgeable and experienced around. When you become a ward manager, you are that more knowledgeable and experienced person. There is no one for you to turn to.

You have more pressure than many non-clinical managers. You are responsible for ensuring that sick and vulnerable people get appropriate care and treatment 24 hours a day, 7 days a week. Everyone, including your team, the patients and their relatives, have very high expectations of you. It's an incredibly responsible job and there are few who would not buckle under the pressure at times. The key is to look after yourself and set up your own support system.

SET UP A PEER SUPPORT GROUP OR ACTION LEARNING SET

The ward manager's job is a lonely one but it needn't be. For some reason, ward managers rarely get together apart from formal sisters' meetings, yet often the best source of support is from others who do the same job and therefore have similar problems.

There is no reason why you cannot set up a small support group of like-minded individuals. It's usually advisable to start off with a small number of around 6 people. Make sure you focus on solutions. Some nurse managers are adept at having lengthy discussions about a problem without ever considering what the solution could be. *Action learning* is a solution-orientated method of learning from each others' problems.

WHAT IS ACTION LEARNING?

Action learning is a process that involves looking at problems from a different perspective, taking action and learning from the result of that action. The idea is that the whole group learns from the actions that the person takes rather than just one person alone. It involves a number of stages:

1. A member of the group presents their problem and the rest of the group listen without interruption.
2. The group encourages further reflection and discussion of the problem using an open and non-biased questioning approach.
3. Following further discussion, the individual together with the group focuses on possible solutions. This enables the individual to devise a plan of action to tackle the problem.
4. After the meeting, the individual goes back to their workplace and follows through the agreed actions.
5. At the following meeting, the individual feeds back to the others what happened as a result of their actions. Together they discuss whether the action worked and what they learned from the process, i.e. if it happened again, what would they do next time?
6. If the action was not successful, another plan can be devised. The group can learn as much from unsuccessful approaches as they do from successful ones.

For further reading on the subject of action learning and how to get started, see Pedlar (2008).

SUPPORT AND CHALLENGE

Action learning is a simple but very effective method of learning and supporting each other. Ideally, it is good to begin with the help of an experienced facilitator, but it is not essential. If there is no one available within your organisation with the right skills and you do not have the funding for an external facilitator, don't let it stop you setting up some sort of 'peer support group' yourself. As long as you meet regularly, you will be able to help each other learn from your experiences and the actions you take.

The key to the success of your group depends on:

- ensuring all discussions are solution orientated, as opposed to problem orientated
- meeting regularly, at least every month
- ensuring that all discussions remain confidential within the confines of the group
- sticking with the same group members as far as possible to enable you to build up trust in each other
- each member being voluntary, i.e. wanting to take part and actively contribute.

The group members need to be able to build up trust and confidence together to be able to challenge each other to think differently about things. Joint reflection with other ward managers is an ideal way of helping you become more effective in your role. It offers the chance to give and receive feedback, which you may not get in such an isolated position. The team you manage will give you a certain amount of feedback but they do not fully understand your issues, having never been in the role themselves. Your line manager's feedback is also limited in that they are working at a distance and in an entirely different role.

DEVELOP THE ROLE OF YOUR DEPUTY

The deputy ward manager(s) can be among your greatest assets. Your aim should be to enable them to develop the skills and ability to do your job within 2 years of being in their current post.

'ACTING UP' IN YOUR ABSENCE

When you take annual leave, you should be able to do so in the knowledge that your ward is in safe hands. You need to be confident that any crises will be dealt with, all your e-mails will be sorted and hopefully you will not have to return to work that has accumulated while you were away. The only way to do this is to prepare your deputy. Help them to develop the skills to 'act up' in your absence.

To prepare your deputy for this role, make sure that you share everything with them. They should be familiar with all aspects of your job. Take them along to meetings so that they are knowledgeable about the groups to which you belong and will be able to represent you in your absence. Don't ask them to replace you at a regular meeting when you have not familiarised them with the process beforehand;

it would be unfair. They need to feel confident to speak up on your behalf. If you are just interested in getting the information, send your apologies. There is no need to waste your deputy's time. Read the minutes instead on your return.

DELEGATE TO IMPROVE SKILLS

Make sure your deputy has some responsibility for aspects of your role such as parts of the budget, investigating complaints or writing reports on your behalf. Delegate early and support them through the process. Don't just show them how to do it. Help them to learn by doing it themselves.

Assign your deputy to deal with your e-mails when you are on 'days off'. You can do this by giving 'proxy access' using their password. It serves to give an insight into your responsibilities. Ensure they have the authority to deal with them as they see fit. Give feedback (not criticism) on your return so they can identify what they did right and wrong and learn a better way of doing things if appropriate.

Don't 'dump' tasks you don't like. Your deputy will come to resent this and it does not help their learning. Stick to delegating tasks that will assist in their learning and development. Don't feel that you must learn something first before your deputy can take it on. If you do not know how to do something, then learn together with your deputy.

Try not to be put out when you find that members of your team prefer to approach your deputy with issues rather than you. It usually has nothing to do with your management style or approachability. People tend to abide by the old hierarchical rules, i.e. go to the person of the next grade, not two grades up. They are just respecting your authority.

ENSURE THEY GET APPROPRIATE SUPPORT

Make sure your deputy has access to a good senior mentor from elsewhere in the hospital. This will enable them to gain an external and thus more objective view on issues at work. A more experienced ward manager from another ward would make a good mentor for them. Your way is not always the only way, so having an external mentor will encourage them to get a different viewpoint, and bring in extra ideas.

Encourage your deputy to join or set up a peer support group or action learning set. They also need an outlet in which to be able to discuss issues and learn from their experiences and mistakes in a safe environment with others who are in similar roles.

WORK ON THEIR STRENGTHS

Your deputy will probably have strengths that differ from yours. Use this to your advantage. If you are not good at presentations, for example, but your deputy excels at them, ensure it is your deputy who gives presentations at important events.

When you undertake a managerial task in the presence of your deputy, such as dealing with aggressive relatives, discuss your performance afterwards. Identify together which aspects went well and which aspects did not go well. By doing this, you are enabling them to learn from your strengths.

Don't feel threatened if your deputy picks things up quickly and performs better than you in certain tasks. Your job is not at risk. Use the situation to your advantage. Their success is a reflection of your efforts. Your own job is made easier. Having a good deputy takes a huge weight off your own shoulders. It helps you to have peace of mind when you are away from the ward for any length of time.

GET YOURSELF A MENTOR

Having a mentor not only helps to achieve the objectives in your personal development plan but will also help in your day-to-day practice by giving you support and guidance or pointing you in the direction of someone who can help. It's advisable to find someone with the right position and experience to enable you to build your confidence in the role. If you are ambitious, a good mentor will also help you further your career.

Don't confuse a managerial mentor with the role of the mentor in nurse education. The role of the mentor in the world of management is totally different from the role of the mentor as advocated by health faculties.

Mentoring in nurse education

In nursing, the term mentor is used to denote the role of the nurse, midwife or specialist community public health nurse who facilitates learning, supervises and assesses students (both pre- and post-registration) in the practice setting (Nursing and Midwifery Council 2008). Formal assessment and paperwork is associated with the role.

Mentoring in management

Mentors for managers should be more experienced managers but *not* the individual's line manager. They usually meet regularly but do not work together in the same department. The relationship is more informal and no formal records are required. It's a bit like clinical supervision except that the supervisor is an experienced manager rather than an experienced clinician. Managerial mentors may also introduce you to their networks so that you can broaden your horizons and become more politically aware.

Most senior managers within health care are familiar with the latter definition of the mentor role. Mentoring at managerial level is seen as a two-way process, in that it enables the senior managers to gain an insight into general issues at the clinical level. Like the clinical supervisor, the role of the mentor in management is to:

● offer a different and objective view of the issues you wish to discuss
● offer a non-judgemental relationship
● develop your skills of reflection to enable you to continually learn from your experiences
● advise, guide, support and help you to solve problems
● help widen your network to give you more of an insight into the politics of the wider organisation.

What a mentor in management won't do is:

- carry out any form of formal assessment
- sort out all your problems for you
- tell you what to do
- offer clinical advice.

Don't choose a mentor because they are 'nice' or you happen to know them. Find someone who can help you reach the goals in your personal development plan. If, for example, you wish to develop your skills in dealing with patient complaints and writing response letters, the complaints manager or one of the non-executive directors who is involved with the complaints department would make an appropriate mentor. As mentioned previously (see p. 171), non-executive directors can make ideal mentors.

HOW TO APPROACH PROSPECTIVE MENTORS

It is not easy to approach someone you don't know and ask them to be your mentor. One option is to shadow them first. Shadowing a senior experienced manager is becoming the 'in' thing to do for managers. If the day turns out well and you feel it would be beneficial, you can then ask them to be your mentor. Otherwise, thank them for their time and find someone else.

PEOPLE TO AVOID AS MENTORS

Be careful about who you choose to be your mentor. There is no point in wasting your time having someone who cannot devote the time and effort to the role. This includes managers who:

- are new to the job and therefore 'finding their feet'
- are not respected within the organisation
- have little influence within your organisation
- are always busy
- have achieved little in their role.

And one last tip is to ensure your line manager knows who your mentor is. It can be quite disconcerting to learn that you have formed a professional relationship with someone who is senior to them. Some managers will need reassuring that the liaison is to improve your skills, not to 'tell tales' about them.

CHOOSE CAREFULLY WHO YOU TALK TO AND WHAT YOU SAY

MEMBERS OF YOUR TEAM

Try not to turn to members of your staff for support. Although you will work together as a team and hopefully have some good times together, it is not wise to use them as a sounding board for any problems you face. If you do, it may make things difficult for you in the future. It could result in:

- your future judgement of that person being affected
- difficulties in dealing with any future inappropriate behaviour
- resentment among those who see one of their colleagues as 'teacher's pet'.

If you are frustrated, angry or upset because of a situation either at work or at home, talk to your mentor, clinical supervisor or your spouse, just not anyone from your team.

YOUR LINE MANAGER

Be careful when talking to your line manager about your problems and frustrations. Always keep in the back of your mind that this person undertakes your appraisals and they or their colleagues may even interview you for future posts. Whether you like it or not, your line manager will talk about you with their colleagues so you want to ensure you create the right impression.

Although you may always be honest, reliable and never talk about people behind their backs, not everyone else is the same. Be wary of others and try not to convey anything negative about you for them to discuss with their colleagues.

BE WARY OF THE INFORMAL NETWORK OR GRAPEVINE

You can never be sure who knows who, who is related to whom and what sort of relationships people had before you joined the organisation. The director of nursing could have trained with your line manager and still meet socially. Your ward receptionist may happen to be a good friend and neighbour of the chief executive. The only safe bet is to ensure you never talk negatively about anyone.

GET TO KNOW INFLUENTIAL PEOPLE

When you attend a work gathering such as a meeting, presentation or conference, try not to stick with your peers where you feel safe and comfortable. You already know them and see them regularly. See if there is anyone there that you could meet; perhaps someone who will introduce you to another part of your organisation. Try and make an effort to talk to someone that you don't already know at meetings.

BE CAREFUL WHAT YOU SAY

If you speak in negative tones, the people you talk to will return those negative tones. If you use positive language, people will be positive in return. If you criticise others, you will be criticised. If you gossip about others, they will gossip about you. What you give out is what you will get back. Always think before you speak.

Be careful also of those who try to manipulate you into divulging information, using statements such as 'I hear your line manager has been having problems with the team in ward X'. Never agree with a statement such as this. Reply with something like 'I know nothing of it' or 'Have you talked to her about what you've heard?' Never be drawn into such conversations even if you agree and do not like the way your manager is handling things. Let your manager know how you feel by all means, but never let it be known to others. Disloyalty earns disrespect.

REDUCE STRESS

Stress is a word used very liberally nowadays. Everyone seems stressed. People talk of suffering from the stress of exams, interviews, giving presentations, holding dinner parties, starting a new job, etc. Stress is not something that happens to you. Stress is your *reaction* to something that happens to you. It's 'the adverse reaction people have to excessive pressure or other types of demand placed on them' (Health and Safety Executive 2011). In other words, how you react to the '*excessive pressure*' or '*other types of demand*' determines the amount of stress you feel.

You will always have pressure of some sort or other in your work. A certain amount of pressure is needed to keep you motivated, and we all know about good stress and bad stress, but if it exceeds your capacity to cope, it can make you ill. When you are in the midst of dealing with continual excessive day-to-day demands it can be difficult to recognise the signs. Ask yourself:

- Do you often think at the beginning of the shift 'here we go again'?
- Do you find there are no more good days, just one bad day after another?
- Do you constantly feel that you cannot get things done; that the barriers are too big?
- Do you feel that you simply do not have the energy to do the job any more?
- Do you find that you are always busy, doing too many jobs at once, trying to be available to everyone?
- Do you take increasing amounts of work home with you and/or does thinking about work keep you awake at night?
- Do you find it more difficult to switch off, even on your 'days off'?
- Are you taking too much comfort in food or alcohol?
- Do you increasingly suffer with continual aches and pains, a tight stomach or indigestion?
- Do you increasingly suffer from frequent colds and infections?
- Do you feel more anxious than you used to?

It is important to recognise the symptoms of stress. These are just a sample. If you allow them to persist, you are risking serious health problems.

COPING WITH THE PRESSURE

The job you are doing is inherently stressful. After all, you have an extremely responsible job. It is normal and healthy to feel stressed on some days, and you will have good and bad days. It is not normal when you are stressed every day and there are no more good days. If you do find things are just getting on top of you, then it is a good idea to stop and think if there are different ways of doing the job or ways of coping with its inherently stressful nature. These include the following:

1. Going to see your manager to identify and agree areas where your workload can be reduced (see Ch. 2).
2. Identifying areas for further training and development to enable you to deal with certain pressures.
3. Setting up a group with your peers to support and learn from each others' experiences.
4. Having a mentor or clinical supervisor to help you deal with difficult situations and learn from them.
5. Thinking about your own health and lifestyle.

THINK ABOUT YOUR OWN LIFESTYLE

You should also think about the way you are leading your life right now. Do you have

● poor health habits (e.g. smoking, consuming too much processed food and fizzy drinks)?
● negative attitudes and feelings (e.g. dwelling on mistakes, thinking everyone else is right)?
● unrealistic expectations (e.g. expecting all staff to know everything and work as hard as you do)?
● perfectionism (e.g. expecting work to be completed to the same standard even when adequate staffing or resources are not available)?

LOOK AFTER YOUR HEALTH

You need to be in the best of health to be alert enough to make the right decisions and support your staff. Hospitals are hot, humid places and you are on your feet all day. If you do not drink water regularly throughout your shift you will suffer from symptoms of dehydration. These include lack of concentration, irritability and headaches and not necessarily just a feeling of thirst. If you do not find the time to eat properly at work, you may find yourself compensating when you get home. It's not a healthy habit to get into. If you make time at work to eat and drink sufficiently you will not only be more alert and productive at work, you may also have some energy left for when you get home. In addition, you are exposed to many varieties of viruses and bacteria at work, so need to ensure that you are in good physical health to prevent you succumbing to illness.

If you decide to work some nights as well, you have to be particularly attentive to your health, as well as the health of your staff who do regular internal rotation. Some tips on remaining healthy during night shifts based on a literature review by Horrocks and Pounder (2006) include:

● taking a 2-hour afternoon nap before your first night
● taking a 30–45 minute nap between 3am and 6am

- eating proper meals (high protein, low carbohydrate appears to be better for maintaining alertness)
- using caffeine cautiously as its effects last up to 4 hours afterwards, so avoid it 4 hours before the end of the night shift. Also, a small dose of caffeine before the 30–45 minute nap may help to increase alertness on waking.

TAKE TIME OFF WHEN YOU ARE ILL

Going to work when you are not fit enough is defined as 'presenteeism', and is particularly widespread among those who work longer hours within the NHS (Boorman 2009).

It used to be generally accepted that the body needs time to rest during illness and time to recuperate afterwards. In the past, if you were ill you took time off work to allow your body to 'fight' the illness, and an extra few days to ensure that you were fit enough for return. Nowadays it seems to be accepted that you should work through the illness. Hodgkinson (2005) illustrates this exceedingly well by describing the Lemsip adverts through the ages. These originally focused on the 'steaming cup of smooth nectar' which was 'part of the delicious and much-needed slow down that illness can bring into our life'. Nowadays their adverts, like many others, focus on getting us through the day. Take a pill. 'No time to be ill. No time for bed. Go, go, go.'

If you are ill, your body needs time to recuperate. Your health is more important than your job. In addition, going to work with an infectious illness (i.e. a cold) really is not wise, particularly when you are infecting sick, vulnerable patients. Try and set an example for your staff. If you have a nasty cold or flu, stay at home.

GET OVER MISTAKES AND MOVE ON

> Success is the result of good judgement.
> Good judgement is the result of experience.
> Experience is often the result of bad judgement.
> (Robbins 2001: 34)

Don't dwell on things. In any job you will make mistakes; it's all part of the learning process. It is so easy to feel pressured when you have made a mistake, particularly in the clinical environment where patient care may have been compromised. The worry over a poor clinical decision, the distress from having upset people or the anguish of feeling you have let the side down can be overwhelming, if you allow it to be.

Try and deal with your mistakes in the following three stages:

1. Take corrective action and/or ask for help as appropriate.
2. Talk it through with someone (individual or group) and learn from it.
3. Take action to reduce the risk of you making the same mistake again.

The key is to be open and honest. Never cover up, always talk it through with someone and learn from it. If you allow yourself to continually worry about your mistakes, it will increase your stress levels and gradually affect your health and self-esteem.

BE WARY OF PERFECTIONISM

Are you a perfectionist? Perfectionists tend to get more upset when under pressure and are more likely to cover up mistakes than others. They are also less likely to ask for help. Excessive worry over mistakes puts perfectionists at risk of developing mood disorders and even phobias (Kawamura and Frost 2004). If you have tendencies towards perfectionism or are a perpetual worrier, you need to work on changing your mindset. Even if you have compromised patient care, don't let the worry take over your life. Learn from the experience.

Discuss your mistake with your peer support group and let others learn from the experience too. Experience is built on mistakes. If you allow your mistake to make you think and feel negatively, you will become reluctant to try new things. Treat mistakes as learning opportunities.

BE CONFIDENT

Don't feel sorry for yourself and make statements like 'it's all my fault' or 'if only I hadn't done this or that'. You are a manager and need to set an example to others. Talking about yourself like this will not only erode your own self-esteem, it will reduce respect from others. Be honest and say something like 'Sorry about that. It was my decision and with hindsight I accept it was not appropriate. I guess the best thing to do now is …'

DEALING WITH MISTAKES – CHANGING THE CULTURE

Most health care policies and strategies are now focused on being open and honest. Things have gradually been changing since the publication of an important document way back in 2000 entitled *An Organisation with a Memory* (Department of Health 2000), which looked into how the NHS learns from errors and adverse events. A national reporting system was set up to record mistakes, adverse incidents and near misses and to make sure that lessons are learned and people are not punished. The aim was to promote a blame-free culture, which encouraged people in the health service to report mistakes without fear of reprimand. Only in the year 2000, for the first time in its 50-year history, the NHS began to develop a structured universal system to learn from mistakes.

However, changing the structure of the system is the easy part; changing the culture takes a lot longer. Changing the mindset of people working in the NHS after 50 years of punishing people for mistakes is no easy task. There are still some health care managers who continue to perpetuate a 'blame culture'. Nurses today still may not feel entirely comfortable with sharing information when they have made an error, particularly one that has resulted in harm to a patient.

You can help by being a role model. Show your staff that you learn from your mistakes. Help them to discuss and learn from their errors. Create an environment where they can admit and learn from their mistakes without being under threat of punishment or blame. Remember that root cause analysis investigations should investigate the system(s) that led to the error, not the person(s). Don't ever allow it to be otherwise.

REMEMBER IT'S ONLY A JOB

Don't let yourself succumb to work-related burnout. You are at risk if you regularly:

- work more than 37.5 hours per week
- take work home with you
- come in on your 'days off' for meetings or to catch up with things
- think about work when you are not there
- allow staff to call you at home
- cancel days off or annual leave because of work commitments.

If you are allowing any of the above to happen regularly then you are investing too much in your job and not enough in other areas of your life. Take action now. It is your choice. Take stock and think about what you can do and what you will do to ensure that you lead a more balanced and fulfilling life rather than putting all your energies into work.

People who suffer from burnout often blame their jobs, but that isn't necessarily the case. It could be because they have invested too much into their jobs and not enough into other aspects of their lives. The first step is to prioritise your workload to fit into 37.5 hours per week (see Ch. 2). The next step is to review what your priorities are outside of work. These could include getting exercise on a regular basis, seeing more of your family, spending evenings out with friends, taking up or renewing an old hobby. You have to find that balance.

Plan to take some annual leave every 3–4 months and book it at the beginning of the financial year. Don't save it up; spread it throughout the year to give yourself regular breaks. Avoid the 'if only' way of thinking:

- 'If only we had more staff ...'
- 'If only I could get on top of all this paperwork ...'
- 'If only the roster didn't take me so long ...'

Don't prolong getting your life in balance by waiting for all the 'if onlys'. You could be waiting a very long time! Don't let life pass you by. Enjoy the journey not just the destination.

The reason why you are in your job should hopefully be because you gain job satisfaction. If you are not satisfied in your role, it is up to you to make some changes. If not, there is always the option of leaving and moving to a different job, even if you resort to doing some agency work for a time. Sometimes, a break serves to allow you to stand back and take a look at your life, think about what you enjoy and what you really want to do. Put yourself first, not your job.

ACTION POINTS

- Get a group of five or six other ward managers together and set up an action learning group to learn from each other.
- Focus on developing the skills of your deputy so they can fully support you in your role, especially in your absence.
- Think about getting yourself a mentor or clinical supervisor.
- If you are under too much pressure at work and feeling stressed, identify possible solutions and take action.
- Take steps to ensure that looking after your own health is a priority, including taking sick leave when you are not fit for work.
- Focus on learning from your mistakes rather than worrying about them.
- Ensure you have a competent and confident team behind you by encouraging staff to be open and learn from their own and each other's mistakes
- Book some annual leave to take every 3–4 months. Work to live; don't live to work.

References

Boorman, S., 2009. NHS health and well-being review: interim report. HMSO, London. Online. Available: http://www.dh.gov.uk/prod_consum_dh/groups/dh_digitalassets/documents/digitalasset/dh_108910.pdf Feb 2012.

Department of Health, 2000. An organisation with a memory. HMSO, London. Online. Available: http://www.dh.gov.uk/assetRoot/04/08/89/48/04088948.pdf Feb 2012.

Health and Safety Executive, 2011. What is stress? Online. Available: http://www.hse.gov.uk/stress/furtheradvice/whatisstress.htm Feb 2012.

Hodgkinson, T., 2005. How to be idle. Penguin, London.

Horrocks, N., Pounder, R., 2006. Working the night shift: preparation, survival and recovery. A guide for junior doctors. Royal College of Physicans, London.

Kawamura, K., Frost, R.O., 2004. Self-concealment as a mediator in the relationship between perfectionism and psychological distress. Cognitive Therapy and Research 28, 183–191.

Nursing and Midwifery Council, 2008. Standards to support learning and assessment in practice. NMC, London. Online. Available: http://www.nmc-uk.org/Publications/Standards/ Feb 2012.

Pedlar, M., 2008. Action learning for managers. Gower, Hampshire.

Robbins, A., 2001. Notes from a friend. Pocket Books, London.

BE A GOOD ROLE MODEL

A good manager sets standards concerning the way their staff and patients should be treated. A major part of your role is to set an example for your staff to follow by showing them:

● how you can cut through bureaucracy to make things happen
● how you expect them to conduct themselves
● how you expect them to treat the patients.

Behaviour is highly contagious. Few of us have spent time with a friend in a low mood and not felt a lowering of our own mood as a result. The way you behave has a huge effect on how your team behave. Always bear that in mind.

BE SMART

Where expression of feelings and attitudes are concerned, it has been found that 55% of the impression we make on others is determined by what they see, 38% by what they hear and 7% by the words we use (Mehrabian 1981). In other words, people are very much influenced by how you look and sound, a lot more than by what you say.

Appearance counts; there is no doubt about it. Just because you have a set uniform, it does not mean that you do not have to bother with what you look like. The image you present to others at work will be seen as a reflection of your level of confidence and self-esteem. The way you control your posture and use your body language can persuade others that you are more or less confident than you might actually be feeling that day.

UNIFORM POLICY

Make a point of adhering strictly to your organisation's uniform policy. If you deviate in any way at all, it gives the green light for others in your team to do so. You may think that wearing a personalised wristband is fine, for example, but if it flouts the uniform policy it is not fine. If you wear one, then you would not be able to reprimand staff for wearing chains around their necks or not tying back long hair.

Don't blame the system if you have only been given two uniforms and therefore cannot keep them clean. You are the manager; it's up to you to cut through the bureaucracy and get yourself and your team the required number of uniforms each.

SET THE STANDARD WITH YOUR OWN UNIFORM

1. Make sure your uniform is clean and stain-free (and fits properly).
2. Make sure your shoes are clean and/or polished. Many people consider scruffy shoes to be a bad reflection on the wearer.
3. Remove all extra jewellery. Wearing items such as a wristwatch instead of a fobwatch will give your team members the opportunity to start wearing extra bits of jewellery too. It's unhygienic, unprofessional and a health and safety hazard. Don't encourage it.
4. Ensure that you have a name badge which displays your job title prominently. Use only the title of ward manager, sister or charge nurse. All other titles are not generally recognisable by the public.

PERSONAL GROOMING

Personal grooming should also be in tip-top condition:

1. Don't neglect your hands and nails. Antiseptic handwash, alcohol gel and the constant use of paper towels can play havoc with your skin. Keep a small tube of hand cream in your pocket. Keep your nails short.
2. Keep your hair neat and tied up if long. Your hairstyle can soften or sharpen your image. You will look less confident if you hide behind your hair or have straggly bits hanging over your face.
3. For women, be sparing with make-up.
4. If you smoke, camouflage the smell when you return to the ward. Use mints and wash your hands. The smell is very distinctive and can be off-putting for non-smokers. It can also exacerbate nausea in sick patients.
5. Be professional at all times. When you are on non-uniform days such as awaydays, meetings or office days, continue to dress smartly. A manager can take no days off from being smart. Your appearance is the most noticeable thing about you.

Some feel that it is unfair to judge people on their appearance but when you meet many people for a few minutes each day (i.e. patients, relatives, senior managers, other health care professionals), they do not have the time to get to know the 'real' you. Like it or not, they will be influenced largely by how you present yourself.

MAKE A GOOD FIRST IMPRESSION

First impressions are powerful and permanent. You never get a second chance to make a good first impression. People form an opinion within the first few seconds of meeting you so it is important to get your image right with all new acquaintances.

VISITORS TO THE WARD

Show your staff the way you would like all visitors to be greeted. Everyone in your team should take the initiative in making people feel welcome. Don't allow your staff to continue writing at the main desk while visitors wait to speak. Their reticence to address the visitor may be considered as rude and intimidating. It will leave a lasting first impression that will colour future contacts with that visitor and your team.

Ensure all your staff wear proper name badges. The enormous array of uniforms and job titles in health care today make it extremely confusing for people to work out who's who and who does what. While they are not a substitute for a personal introduction, they do help visitors recognise who people are.

NEW MEMBERS OF STAFF

Make it your aim to greet all new members to the team. Starting a new job is a daunting experience. Having someone come over, introduce themselves, shake your hand and ask how you are is a very welcoming experience and one that is often not forgotten. New junior doctors become future consultants and GPs. Student nurses may well go on to become future nurse managers with whom you will liaise. Those first impressions of being on your ward will stay with them.

CENTRE THE SPOTLIGHT ON THE OTHER PERSON

The key to making a good first impression is to centre the spotlight on the other person. Demonstrate immediately that they are the centre of the conversation. This is particularly pertinent in the case of patients and their relatives. They are not there to hear about you; they want to feel confident that they have your full attention and that you are in control. Think how you would feel as a relative presented with the following greeting:

'Oh hello. We are a bit busy at the moment. I'm afraid that your father's admission was unexpected. We are a little short staffed but I promise I will come over and see you as soon as I can.'

This greeting is focused on the person who is making it and creates the impression that they are not in control of things. If you focus your greeting on the other person, it creates a far better first impression:

'Hello there. Your father has been admitted to bed ten. If you'd like to take a seat in the dayroom, I'll come and explain everything to you in about 20 minutes once we've settled him in.'

Visitors do not need to know all about your problems. They need to be reassured that their relatives are in a safe environment and cared for by competent professionals.

The same applies when you are meeting other health professionals:

Focus on self: 'Hello. I'm the ward sister. I've been here for a good few years and know how the place runs like the back of my hand. If you need anything, let me know.'

Focus on other person: 'Hello. You must be Mark Smith. I understand you've just started. How are you settling in?'

While both greetings are perfectly acceptable, the latter example demonstrates that if you focus your greeting on the other person it can help them to feel a lot more comfortable and relaxed. Using the name of a new acquaintance also makes it more personal.

Focus also on listening to what the other person has to say. You'll make a good initial impression if you demonstrate good listening skills. Give positive verbal cues such as 'that's useful to know' or 'what happened next?' Try not to take over by giving unsolicited advice or relating a similar experience; this only serves to refocus the conversation on to you. Aim to listen to your new acquaintance, not to make them listen to you. It also helps if you maintain steady eye contact. Don't be constantly looking over their shoulder thinking about what you should be doing next. Try not to interrupt by answering the telephone or busying around doing other things.

Giving a good first impression gets you off to the right start and will save a lot of time and effort later on. The benefits far outweigh the inconvenience of dedicating a few minutes of your time.

ALWAYS SMILE AND BE POSITIVE

Your facial expressions affect the mood of your team. If you look gloomy and depressed, it is not only unattractive, it will make others feel gloomy and depressed too. Yet when you smile at someone, they will feel happier in an instant; few people would not smile back. It makes people warm to you.

Try and smile even in the face of adversity. However, do make sure it is genuine. People who put on a smile all the time without being genuinely happy can be irritating. If you are not happy and cannot smile, do something positive about it. Being deliberately positive increases the mood in both you and your team. Smile to yourself now and notice how it increases your mood. Smiling makes you feel happier; feeling happier makes you smile!

Be aware that your facial expressions and body language affect the way the people around you feel and the way they work. This ultimately affects the standard of patient care. A positive attitude produces a good working atmosphere. It not only increases morale, it leads to increased performance and job satisfaction. Search for opportunities to invest in each person who works for you. See each interaction with a member of your team as an opportunity to increase their positivity.

BE OPTIMISTIC

Being consistently optimistic is a prerequisite for great leaders. You do not have to be a born leader to have this attribute; it can be learned. Start thinking positively and tell yourself that things are going to be good today. Act like things are going well and before long you may even start believing it yourself.

When people ask you how you are, don't reply 'oh, not so bad really' or 'can't grumble'. When people ask this question, they are usually only being polite and not asking how you really are. Smile and be positive. Use phrases like, 'I'm good' or 'I'm very well indeed. How are you?' Being upbeat is infectious.

FOCUS ON THE SOLUTION, NOT THE PROBLEM

Present solutions. There is usually something positive in any situation; you just need to draw it out. If you are greeted with a statement such as 'We are three staff down today and there are no agency available; how on earth are we going to cope?', don't let your facial expression fall with a reply like 'Oh no, I don't believe it'. Keep smiling, be positive and say something like 'Right, we'll have to make a list together of the tasks that we we will leave undone, so that the patients are safe.''

Associate yourself with people who make you feel good. If your manager is one of those people whose glass is always half empty, listen and learn. Experiences with managers like this help you learn. Watch the effect that they are having. You'll see first hand how negativity breeds negativity. Strive to ensure you do not emulate such habits.

Luckily, the attributes of great leaders can be developed by anyone who is passionate and committed in their work. Start today by being cheerful, smiling and optimistic if you can, no matter what the situation you are in.

SPEAK CLEARLY

Your speaking style conveys more about you than maybe you would wish. People determine your intelligence, education, even your leadership ability by the words you use and by how you say them. The whole reason for speaking is to impart information clearly and effectively. If you tend to speak too softly or mumble, it could result in:

- others not being able to hear or understand you
- being misheard or misunderstood
- giving the impression that you lack confidence
- giving the impression that you don't really have anything interesting to say and so are insignificant. As a result, people will quickly forget you.

If you stand upright with confidence, make eye contact and speak clearly, people will assume that you are knowledgeable and have something specific to say which is relevant to them. They will remember you.

FOCUS ON YOUR PRONUNCIATION

The nature of your role means you have to be able to think fast and make quick decisions throughout your shift. For some health workers, this comes out in their speech. It is a natural tendency to talk quickly when pressured or stressed. Speaking too quickly means that people cannot keep up with you and there is a tendency to 'fall over' your words. The result is that not all of your message will get through. Some find it happens more often towards the end of the shift. Focusing on your pronunciation is a good way of slowing down your speech. People will be more attentive and more likely to understand what you are saying without having to ask you to repeat it or glazing over and stopping bothering to listen.

Concentrate on how you pronounce your words. Some people get into the habit of dropping the 'g's and 't's from the end of their words. This results in words being slurred together and can make you come across as uneducated. Say the following sentences out loud as if you were talking to one of your colleagues at work:

- 'Are you going to start the ward round in a minute?'
- 'Do you want to start taking your breaks now?'
- 'I'll sort out the discharge arrangements if you just take this phone call?'

Did you articulate each syllable and pronounce all the 'g's and 't's? Be aware that not doing so can inhibit you getting your message across clearly.

Filler phrases such as 'you know', 'actually' or lots of 'um's and 'er's also distract people from listening to what you are saying. People will notice these repetitive phrases more than they notice what you are saying. Lazy, sloppy speech indicates a lack of commitment and energy, and even arrogance. It can be construed that you don't care and you can't be bothered. This is not an image you want to portray, nor one you want others to copy.

YOUR TELEPHONE MANNER

The way you answer the telephone speaks volumes about you. Saying something like 'Ward 10?' is really not sufficient. 'Ward 10, Sister speaking' is an improvement, but 'Ward 10, Sister speaking. How may I help you?' is more warm and welcoming. It also makes you come across as confident and professional.

Body language is extremely important. The way you stand and the way you speak affects your total image. If you are constantly fidgeting or looking anywhere but at the person you are speaking to, you will appear ill at ease. This affects your telephone manner too. If you are slouched across the desk talking to someone over the phone, you will come across as less controlled than if you sit upright.

STOP APOLOGISING

Be wary about apologising before you speak, and if you do tend to do this, try and break the habit unless you have genuinely done something to be sorry about. It can come across as if you are apologising for your presence and people are quick to pick up on that. Take the following examples:

- 'Sorry to bother you, would you mind taking one of our patients to theatre?'
- 'Sorry. I can see you are busy but Dr Smith has come to see Mrs Jones.'

If you find yourself using phrases such as those outlined above, try using the following alternative approaches:

- 'We have a patient ready for theatre. Is anyone available?'
- 'Excuse me interrupting you. Dr Smith is here to see Mrs Jones.'

These things may seem minor, but the way you convey yourself is so important if you want to be taken seriously.

And one last tip: swearing is not appropriate for someone in a managerial role. It is not only unprofessional but some consider that people who swear are of lower intelligence. It is often seen as a sign that someone's vocabulary is inadequate. When used *very* sparingly, it can have a powerful effect and make people take notice, but when used regularly, it will lower people's opinion of you and sets a bad example.

BE RELAXED AND IN CONTROL

If you are smart, articulate, always smiling and positive in your outlook, you will come across as warm, friendly and confident. In other words, you are creating the impression that you are in control; your work does not control you. Walk upright (no rounded shoulders) and greet people with a good strong handshake. It's an attractive quality; people are drawn to attractiveness.

KEEP YOUR COOL

Never lose your temper. Loss of temper means loss of control. By all means, say how you feel but ensure you remain cool, calm and collected as you do so. There is nothing wrong with saying, 'I know you have a job to do, but I find your attitude quite impossible' and walking away if necessary. Don't get into a heated argument. It is unbecoming of a senior manager and will be talked about for years to come by the other party and any onlookers.

MANAGE CONFLICT WITH CONFIDENCE

It helps in times of conflict if you can identify whether you and the other party are adopting a parent, child or adult state. Eric Berne (a psychoanalyst who wrote the best-selling book called *Games People Play*) puts forward the theory that people tend to take on the persona of a parent, adult or child depending on what situation they are in (Berne 1968). In times of conflict, try and decipher what role you are playing:

Parent state: Are you nurturing the other person by trying to give advice or protect them by not giving enough responsibility? Are you being critical perhaps by telling them off for breaking the rules?
Child state: Are you feeling insecure and expecting to be told what to do? Are you trying to rebel against 'the rules'?
Adult state: Are you being sensible, calm and logical? Are you able to keep your emotions from interfering with the situation?

According to Berne, there is no 'best' or 'worst' state. Each can be helpful if used in the right situation. Being in 'adult mode' all the time can make for a very boring person. However, having an awareness of what state you and the other person are in can help you manage relationships more effectively.

Situations of conflict can be resolved by concentrating on bringing both parties into 'adult state'. If, for example, you have some members of your team who decide that they can behave how they like with complete disregard about the effects they have on others, you may be tempted to take on the role of the controlling parent.

This can exacerbate the situation, whereas if you take on the adult role, which tends to be more unemotional and detached, it could help diffuse the situation and help produce a matching adult state in others.

USE OF EMPATHY

Use of empathy is often a good way of resolving the situation if someone is being difficult. Being empathic means showing that you understand the other person's point of view by using phrases such as 'I understand what you are saying; I get frustrated with the system too sometimes'. Self-disclosure also helps. Tell them how their behaviour makes you feel, such as 'Your tone is making me feel uncomfortable'.

When you are in a situation of conflict, try and match the other person's parent or child state by empathising with them, then move them into more of an adult state by suggesting a joint solution. Using 'we' rather that 'you' or 'I' also helps in diffusing heated situations. This is illustrated in the following example:

> *Manager*: 'I'm not happy about the way you run the ward. You should not allow staff to be drinking coffee at the main reception desk.' *(Angry critical parent mode.)*
> *Sister*: 'I can understand why you think like that. I feel the same myself at times.' *(Use of empathy and self-disclosure.)* 'The problem is when we are short staffed, the staff are unable to leave the ward for their breaks. Perhaps we could come up with an alternative solution?' *(Sensible adult mode, suggesting joint solution.)*

Whatever you do, always keep your cool. Working in health care, we are all subject to chronic staff shortages, bed pressures, poor resources and relentless performance targets. No wonder working relationships are constantly put under strain. Some would say that conflict is inevitable, but if you keep your cool it does not have to be.

Further tips that may help in times of adversity include:

1. Always manage difficult people face-to-face. Leaving voice-mail, e-mail, fax, notes, etc. will only serve to increase their animosity.
2. Control your own emotions; do not get angry and shout back. If you feel threatened or intimidated, say that you will leave and come back later when things have calmed down. Put some time and distance between the two of you. Never walk out in a huff.
3. Notice those in your team who are not being difficult, those who work hard and without complaint. Reward them. Just a simple thank you may be all that is needed. Don't allow the difficult ones to claim most of your attention.

MAKE YOUR WRITING DISTINGUISHABLE

How you write is very important. You will be judged not only on what you write but also on how your writing looks. If members of your staff see that you write scruffily on patient documentation, they will not bother to be neat and tidy either. If you don't bother to refer to the care plan when writing your evaluations, your staff will not bother either. You set the standard in everything you do, so don't let your writing let you down.

HANDWRITING

Using a distinctive pen, a fountain pen, for example, will show out on documentation. Take the time to ensure that everything you write is:

- neat and legible
- large and noticeable
- consistent.

Make sure that your staff notice your handwriting. When they recognise it, they will notice the content. Your aim is for them to see your high standards of documentation.

In law, the clinical record portrays the standard of care. You should demonstrate a high standard of care at all times. Remember that patients' records are also reviewed by an array of health professionals – anaesthetists, surgeons, physiotherapists, complaints managers and even solicitors. They will all judge the standard of care based on the standard of your records.

CARE PLANS AND EVALUATIONS

Unfortunately, the task of writing care plans and evaluations is still often relegated to the end of the shift. This is a time when people are tired and rushing to get everything done so that they can get home. It's not the best time to write such an important document. Demonstrate to your staff that they can make entries throughout the shift. Each time you complete an episode of care or if there is a change in the patient's condition, write an entry in the evaluation section (in your distinguishable handwriting). Obviously it is not possible for you to do this each and every time but try and get into the habit of writing your evaluations and any care plan updates throughout the shift rather than saving them all until the end. This is also recommended in principle 3 of the Record Keeping Guidance (Nursing and Midwifery Council 2010). Make a particular point of doing this when you have a member of staff or student to shadow you for a shift.

At the time of writing, many areas are now switching over to computerised care planning and evaluations. However, there are some areas where the staff write care plans and/or evaluations by hand, then enter the data into a computerised system at the end of the shift (or worse still, delegate the task to the poor night staff!). Use your common sense. Care plans and evaluations should be completed with the involvement of the patient, so if you do not have the resources, i.e. access to a sufficient number of hand-held PCs, continue to use paper-based ones until you do. Or write a business case for extra staff to take on the extra administrative workload!

E-MAILS

E-mails are another area where it is wise to think how you would like others to e-mail you. People will also judge your intellect through the way you write your e-mails. As a general rule:

- Go through your e-mails each day. Answer them quickly, preferably within 24 hours.

- Keep all e-mails short; never more than one screenful or three paragraphs.
- Always make the best use of the subject heading such as 'Re: Impending staffing shortage across medical unit next week' or 'Benchmarking meeting on Monday cancelled'. Subject headings like these mean your e-mails are more likely to be opened and noted.
- Make your e-mails easier to read by writing the most important information in the first paragraph and the background/supporting information in the rest of the e-mail. If you need to send more than one screen of information, try and send it as an attachment instead.
- Never use your work e-mail account for private or personal e-mails. All your e-mails should come as no surprise if another member of your team gains access to them. It is good development for a deputy or someone who is shadowing you for the day to go through your e-mails with you. It helps them to gain a good insight into your role and responsibilities.
- Bear in mind that no e-mail is confidential. If you wish to send a message that is confidential or controversial in any way, use the phone or use face-to-face contact wherever possible.
- Don't send blind copies (bcc) casually. They imply that you are going behind someone's back.
- Don't ask for a receipt unless absolutely necessary. It implies that you do not trust the recipient to read or respond promptly to your e-mails.
- Use the urgent icon sparingly. If not, really urgent e-mails you send in the future may get overlooked.
- Don't use CAPITAL LETTERS. In e-mail language, this is construed as SHOUTING!
- Don't send jokes via e-mail. If you receive them just delete them; do not forward them.
- Always use a positive tone and be aware that the tone of e-mails can be misconstrued.
- Never leave your computer unattended. You don't want your staff or any others sending e-mails to people in your name.

Everything you write, whether by hand or computer, speaks volumes about you. Make sure you are conveying the right image and encourage others to have the same high standards.

BE AWARE OF HOW OTHERS SEE YOU

To be a good role model, you have to know yourself. Hopefully you know your strengths and weaknesses from your own point of view, but are you sure that others see you in the same light as you see yourself? How realistic is your image of yourself?

You may, for example, see one of your strengths as being assertive and getting things done, but others may regard you as aggressive and loud and as a result may shy away from you. You may feel that you are weak at organising your team, whereas your team may see it as a strength that you allow your team to organise their own work and make their own decisions.

ASK PEOPLE TO POINT OUT YOUR KEY STRENGTHS AND WEAKNESSES

A simple way to find out what others think of you is to ask. Some recommend that you ask each of your peers, members of your team and your line manager to write down what they think your three key strengths are and identify one area that could be improved. This can be quite a humbling exercise and some would have difficulty asking their colleagues what they think about them.

ASK PEOPLE ABOUT THEIR WORK SATISFACTION

Another way to find out how you are perceived is to ask people about your leadership skills but to put it to your team in a way that makes it seem like you are asking about their work. One way to do this would be to devise a questionnaire based on one of the many leadership models. One example is Kouzes and Posner (2007) who outlined five behaviours of a good leader:

1. Challenging the process.
2. Inspiring a shared vision.
3. Encouraging the heart.
4. Enabling others to act.
5. Modelling the way.

Think of some questions that would enable you to find out how your behaviour affects your team. Here are some examples.

Challenging the process

'Do you feel we should spend more time and effort on finding different ways of doing things at work?'
'Do you feel that the work of the team could be improved if we looked outside the organisation for more ideas?'
'Do you feel we take the time to learn from our mistakes?'

Inspiring a shared vision

'Do you feel that you are fully aware and involved with what's going on in the ward?'
'Are you excited about working in this ward over the coming year?'
'Do you feel enthusiastic about the future of the ward?'

Encouraging the heart

'Do you feel your work is valued within the team?'
'Do you feel that your work is noticed and appreciated?'
'Are you usually thanked when a job has been done well?'

Enabling others to act

'Do you feel your views are listened to seriously?'

'Do you feel that you have sufficient opportunities to learn new skills in your role?'
'Do you feel that you have enough autonomy in deciding how to go about your work?'

Modelling the way

'Are you comfortable with what the expectations are of you in your job?'
'Do you feel that your team has a good plan with achievable goals about where we are all going?'
'Do you feel well led as a team?'

Make it simple. Don't get them to start grading the answers. You do not have time to collate lots of different answers. Ask members of your team to answer a simple yes or no to each of the questions. The sections that have two or more 'no' answers suggest that you could perhaps improve in that particular area. This is a less threatening way of achieving personal feedback than if you were to ask individuals to identify your strengths and weaknesses.

MAKING USE OF FEEDBACK

If, for example, you have consistent 'no' answers in the section for 'Encouraging the heart', perhaps you need to work on your feedback skills (see p. 49). If you received consistent 'no' answers in the section for 'Inspiring a shared vision', you may want to look at establishing shared goals for your team (see p. 45) and perhaps shadowing someone senior within your organisation for a time to pick up on the skills required to inspire a team.

Make sure you get feedback from as many team members as you can. Don't just pick the 'nice' ones. You may get a biased view or they may complete it in a certain way to try and please you. Try and get the views from a good cross-section of staff within your team. Once you get more confidence, asking individuals what they think your strengths and weaknesses are will give you more specific and individual feedback which you can work on. To be a good leader it is advisable to be aware of what others think of you.

SET AN EXAMPLE WITH YOUR CHOICE OF LANGUAGE

Don't let negative people set the tone. There is always at least one person in a team who will consistently use language such as:

'We can't do that.'
'They'll never allow us to do that.'
'We've tried it all before, it won't work.'
'We've got enough to do.'
'We haven't got enough staff.'
'They don't know what it's like for us.'
'There's nothing we can do.'

These people have the attitude that someone else is always in control. They are not choosing what they do; other people rule their lives. They have a tendency to absolve responsibility for any choices they make.

Think about the language you use:

'I have to go to the sisters' meeting this afternoon.'
'We have to do it this way because …'
'I've tried but it makes no difference.'
'If only we could recruit one more member of staff.'

Using language like this will give the impression you are not in control. Not only that; others will adopt this negative tone. Blaming outside forces for your situation makes you a victim and is hardly the quality required of a good ward manager. Think carefully about the language you use. Make sure others see you as someone who is in control of the situation. Do you *have* to go to that meeting or do you *choose* to go?

Managers will often use negative phrases to cover up their guilt at leaving staff extra work in their absence. Instead, just explain why you have chosen to go to the meeting: 'I shall be leaving you this afternoon for a couple of hours to attend a meeting about the future changes within the directorate'. This is just as acceptable but shows that you are in charge of what you are doing.

Use positive language such as:

'What is the alternative?'
'I will …'
'I choose to …'
'I prefer to …'
'I shall …'
'OK, so that didn't work, what shall we try instead?'
'I have decided to …'
'I am going to …'

It's all in the mind. If you think you are powerless, you will be powerless and others will see you as such. You will start producing every excuse you can to justify why you have to do something or why you cannot do something. It becomes a self-fulfilling prophecy. Change your way of thinking and you change your way of seeing things and the way others see you.

NEVER MOAN OR GOSSIP ABOUT OTHERS

Try and keep negative opinions to yourself. Don't get pulled into a situation where a group of staff sit around talking about individuals who are not present to defend themselves. Retrain yourself to look for the good in each person and in each situation. Change the conversation around by pointing out the positive things about the individual or change the subject completely. If you gossip, your staff will gossip. As their role model, think about what behaviour you are portraying to them.

Moaning and gossiping about others is contagious and achieves nothing. Once one person starts whingeing, others join in and it creates an overall negative atmosphere. Your job is to maintain a continual positive atmosphere. In addition to this, if you do moan and whinge about others, your staff may well think, 'If my manager says this about others, what is said about me when my back is turned?'

People are wary when in the company of gossips and will not talk freely. As a manager, you need to be seen as someone that people can be open and honest with. Being heard gossiping will only hinder you. Never let your guard down, even on social nights out. Socialising with your staff is perfectly acceptable but be careful. Don't get involved in negative conversations about other people at work.

WHY DO PEOPLE GOSSIP AT WORK?

People who spend a lot of time gossiping at work may either be bored with their jobs or haven't got enough responsibility. If it is happening on your ward, perhaps you need to look at how their work is being organised. Staff who spend their time completing a set list of tasks (e.g. washes by 11:00, observations at 12:00) find their work neither challenging nor inspiring. Make sure that neither you nor your staff are delegating tasks like this to their juniors. Empower staff to take on responsibility for the whole patient rather than just tasks. If you encourage your senior staff to take on more responsibilities, they should hopefully take note and encourage their juniors in the same way.

MOANING ABOUT WORK

If you find yourself moaning about work, make yourself think of a solution to the issue instead. If there isn't one, then stop moaning; it only serves to waste time. If there is a solution, put your efforts into solving the issue instead of wasting your valuable time moaning about it. People tend to moan or procrastinate when faced with:

- a large workload
- unrealistic time commitments
- too many interruptions
- work requiring skills they do not have.

If this is happening to your team regularly, perhaps you need to take a step back and look at what you and your team can do to control your workload rather than allowing it to control you (see Ch. 2).

CHANGE THE MOANING CULTURE

If you are one of those people whose glass is more half empty than half full, try and make a conscious effort to look on the bright side. People are much more likely to warm to you if you're talking positively rather than negatively. Get into the habit of it and you'll not only give yourself a lift, but others too.

Make the staff room a nice place to be in by adding things that lift people's spirits. Put photos on the wall from ward nights out. Ensure there are nice mugs for tea rather than drab paper cups. Make sure there is always a plentiful supply of coffee, tea, sugar and milk. Perhaps even get the staff to add an extra £1 to the kitty, and when things are particularly challenging, buy some cream cakes for the team. These may seem small gestures but together they will help to prevent a climate of moaning and gossiping and general dissatisfaction.

DON'T STAGNATE

Demonstrate a personal commitment to improving yourself and others by showing that you are continually willing to learn and develop professionally. Methods you can use to role model that commitment are through:

- sharing your learning and experiences
- involvement in the wider organisation
- involvement in wider professional issues
- having others shadow you.

SHARING YOUR LEARNING AND EXPERIENCES

If you personally attend any courses, teaching sessions or conferences, make a point of sharing what you have learned with the rest of your team. If you have a patient with a condition rarely seen by the team, find out about it and share the knowledge with your team. Don't just encourage others to do this. Show them the way and how it should be done. Your staff will be more willing to share what they have learned with the team if they observe you doing it all the time.

Always practise what you preach. Most nurses remember being told to share their learning as a student or junior staff nurse. It can cause a lot of unnecessary anxiety for them if they are the only ones required to do this. If you and your senior staff put on sessions regularly where you share your learning, it will become common practice and junior staff will be more willing to take part.

INVOLVEMENT IN THE WIDER ORGANISATION

Becoming involved in hospital committees not only widens your networks, it can help your staff to broaden their horizons too. Take one of them along with you to the meetings every now and then to introduce them to the higher 'workings' of the organisation. Show them just how important your meetings are and how they influence clinical practice.

Demonstrating to your staff how influential you are at a higher level gives them an insight as to how influential they can be in their future careers. Give them first-hand knowledge of any decisions made and how and why they will affect future practice. Seeing you have wider influence will increase their respect in your skills and abilities too.

INVOLVEMENT IN WIDER PROFESSIONAL ISSUES

Make sure you are a member or are involved in the professional association linked with your role. If you do not have a specialist association, try other professional bodies. The Royal College of Nursing (RCN) holds various management and leadership forums with which you could become involved. Another option is to join a community group to help develop the links with the community teams.

Don't become involved in any more than two groups at the very most. It would not be appropriate to allow outside commitments to interfere with your day-to-day managerial responsibilities. Make sure also that this commitment is in your work time and recognised as a core responsibility. Some nurses regard work for hospital-wide or professional associations as an extra task that should be done in their own time. That could not be further from the truth. You are furthering the knowledge and expertise of your team. If you elect to do this in your own time, you are conveying the message to your team that you expect them to do that too.

HAVING OTHERS SHADOW YOU

Encourage members of your staff (registered, unregistered and students) to shadow you regularly if you can. Having someone to shadow you will help to keep you up-to-date. They will ask questions and make you think about the way you work. Having to explain why you make decisions stimulates you to think again about why you do things. It's hard work and can be quite challenging but is an enormous benefit to your learning. You can also learn new ideas from those that shadow you. They will be fresh with ideas from other wards where they have worked or with new techniques and knowledge from various courses or study they have undertaken.

Never think you know everything. No matter how long you have been in your job or specialty, there is always more to learn. It is advisable to adopt this attitude at all times. If you still have lots to learn, then your staff will too. If you allow yourself to stagnate, your staff will follow suit.

ACTION POINTS

- Check your uniform policy and make sure you strictly adhere to it as an example to others.
- Make a point of warmly greeting all visitors to your ward and focus the conversation on them.
- Start smiling more and focusing on the positive aspects in all situations.
- Speak slowly, clearly and focus on pronouncing your 'g's and 't's, particularly if you have a tendency to talk quickly.
- In times of conflict, try and identify what state you and the other person are in – parent, child or adult. Use empathy and self-disclosure to bring both into an adult state.
- Buy a pen that will distinguish your writing from others and ensure that everything you write is large, neat and legible.
- Think of ways you can get feedback from your team (in a non-threatening manner) to identify areas you can improve upon.
- Stop yourself each time you say 'I can't' or 'I have to' and change it to 'I will' or 'I choose to'.
- If you have a tendency to gossip or moan about things at work, think about why you do this and what you can do to stop this habit.
- Consider ways in which you can demonstrate to others that you are continually learning by sharing your experiences.

References

Berne, E., 1968. Games people play. Penguin, London.

Kouzes, J., Posner, B., 2007. The leadership challenge, fourth ed. Jossey Bass, San Francisco.

Mehrabian, A., 1981. Silent messages: implicit communication of emotions and attitudes, second ed. Wadsworth, California.

Nursing and Midwifery Council, 2010. Record keeping: guidance for nurses and midwives. Online. Available: http://www.nmc-uk.org/Documents/Guidance/nmcGuidanceRecordKeepingGuidanceforNursesandMidwives.pdf.

MANAGE YOUR MANAGER

A very important, but much neglected, part of being a good manager is building up a good working relationship with your own manager. This may not seem your foremost concern because you are focusing so much on building your own team. But if you make time for your manager, you will ensure that you:

- are more likely to be involved in making important decisions that affect your team
- have greater access to appropriate help to achieve your team's goals

- gain respect and are taken seriously
- learn from your manager's experiences (including mistakes)
- keep well informed
- have greater freedom and authority to act.

If you do not put time and effort into building up a good working relationship with your manager, you can become low on their priority list. This means you could end up having your concerns falling on deaf ears. You may find that they forget to give you information. You could even find that you end up arguing regularly and get labelled as the 'difficult' one.

Having a poor relationship with your manager does you no favours at all. It will hinder your progress. It doesn't matter whether you like them or not; they have access to knowledge and information that you don't. You should find the right ways of working with them to help achieve your goals.

CLARIFY EXPECTATIONS

Problems tend to arise if there is a lack of clarity between you about your tasks and responsibilities.

BE CLEAR ABOUT WHAT YOU EXPECT FROM YOUR MANAGER

You do not have to become great friends with your manager, but you should understand their role and the demands placed on them. If you know what the organisation expects from your manager, then you will understand more readily why they work the way they do and why they make the decisions they do.

Your manager may have a different management style to you. They may be used to giving out orders and telling people what to do rather than involving the team in any decision making. This may not sit well with you. If that is the case, then say so, but don't jump in with both feet. After all, their style may emanate from their own lack of confidence, so to 'attack' them may be counterproductive. Notwithstanding this, try to be clear about your expectations in that you want to be involved, not just informed. Ask your manager for regular feedback, both positive and negative, so that you can continuously improve in your work, rather than wait for your appraisal to find out how you are progressing.

Make sure you get your appraisal each year. Don't wait for your manager to initiate the process. Write down what you want to discuss:

1. Your own self-assessment on how you think you are doing.
2. The objectives you feel are the priorities for your ward.
3. Your personal development needs in order to achieve those objectives.

Forward this information to your manager in preparation for your appraisal. Take control of the process, as you would hope your own staff would do for you. If the meeting is cancelled more than twice, let them know how it makes you feel. Unfortunately, there are still some senior managers who will regularly cancel appraisals (usually only because of disorganisation) without realising the unintended effect it can have on morale.

You need to understand what your manager's own objectives are too. A good manager will ensure that your objectives reflect their own. In that way, you will know that you are both heading in the same direction. It would be detrimental if your objectives were totally different from those of your manager. That would only serve to create tension in your working relationship, not to mention the effect on practice.

Remember that your manager is only human. Sometimes, people are labelled as 'poor' managers because they do not conform to our expectations. Your manager may have become out of touch clinically, for example, but may still be particularly good at helping you to write complaint letters or getting more resources for your ward. Make sure you get the most from what they do well and try not to focus on any weaknesses.

BE CLEAR ABOUT WHAT YOUR MANAGER EXPECTS FROM YOU

Your manager will probably have managed a ward or department before taking promotion. Problems sometimes occur when they expect you to manage your ward in the same way that they did. One of the ways you can ensure that you have full control without interference is to keep your manager fully informed about what you are doing. Show what you are doing well. Be clear about the skills you have and those you want to improve upon. Your manager needs to believe in your abilities before they will trust you.

If your manager does not communicate their expectations clearly, then it is your responsibility to ask what is expected. Your manager may not have good management or support from their own manager; this may affect their own ability to manage you. You need to appreciate their position and accept that perhaps they need prompting to articulate their expectations. Make sure you have what your manager expects in terms of organisational objectives written down clearly during your appraisal. Always refer to these in anything that you do. If your manager comes to you with further projects, ask yourself if it relates to your original objectives. If it does not, question your manager's expectations. Are they perhaps too high?

Try not to get into the habit of propping up a failing or struggling manager. Encourage them to get help and support from elsewhere. You cannot provide your manager with the same support that you give your team. It is not fair on you and you must let them know that.

WORK WITH, NOT AGAINST, YOUR MANAGER

Just because someone is your manager it does not mean that they are perfect and know everything. Like you, they will also be learning from their experiences and mistakes. Don't focus on their weaknesses; nobody is perfect. Focus on their strengths; they would not be in the job if they didn't do something right.

MEET REGULARLY

Have regular meetings to review your objectives. Take the initiative and set up these meetings if your manager does not already do so. The constant changes in health care, including the ever-changing contracts and performance indicators, may result in a need for you to change your priorities. Make sure any changes to priorities are discussed and objectives changed and agreed accordingly. Without keeping a check on them throughout the year, you could find you are going in a different direction to your manager.

REMAIN LOYAL

If you do not like the way your manager works, do something about it. Tell your manager how you feel and suggest ways of changing their approach. Don't complain to others about their way of working. You must be seen to be working on the side of your manager at all times. Disloyal people can never be trusted by both their managers and employees alike. A reputation for disloyalty can be hard to dispel.

PUT A STOP TO ANY INTERFERENCE IN CLINICAL ISSUES

If you feel your manager is interfering too much in clinical issues, it can indicate that they do not have enough confidence in your abilities. You need to ask yourself why. Are you showing them what a good job you do or are you leaving it up to them to find out? Managers do not have time to constantly observe their employees. Take the initiative; keep them abreast of what you do well and any achievements regularly. They will appreciate more of what you do, rather than what you don't do.

Some managers are unable to let go of the clinical side, particularly if they have been promoted internally. Sometimes this means they do not have confidence in their more senior role and are taking refuge in what they do know. The key in this situation is to give consistent positive feedback on what they are doing well; then intersperse this with some feedback about how their additional involvement on the clinical side is affecting you and your team in a non-productive way.

ASSIST IN DECISION MAKING

Some managers find it difficult to decide what to do when confronted with a problem, particularly when clinical skills have become 'rusty'. The best thing you can do in this situation is to help them by outlining the possible solutions, making it clear to them which one you feel is the most suited at that time. You may need to follow this up with clear directions on the steps that need to be taken. Remember always to support them in any decision they make, including the 'fall-out' should it be the wrong decision. Nobody ever wants to hear the phrase 'I told you so' or 'It was the manager's decision, not mine'.

WHAT IF YOUR MANAGER IS ALWAYS TOO BUSY?

Being permanently busy does not mean that more work is getting done. It can sometimes mean the person is not in control of their workload. If your manager is busy and not in control, it will probably affect your work too. Meeting with your manager to confirm what you have defined as your workload (as outlined in Ch. 2) may help them to see that it would be a good idea for them to do the same exercise.

Every time your manager comes to you saying, 'We have to do this ...' (e.g. another audit, a new procedure or a further reduction in staffing levels), ask yourself three very important questions:

1. 'Do we *have* to do this, or do we *choose* to do this?' (if you do not choose to do it, you are not in control), then:
2. 'If we choose not to do this, what will the consequences be?'
3. 'If we choose to do this, how much time and resources will it take, and which of our current tasks will we discontinue in order to make time for the new more important task?'

ACT, IF AN IMPORTANT DECISION HAS BEEN MADE WITHOUT YOUR CONSULTATION

If any important changes need to be made at work, everyone should be consulted. You should be given the chance to say what you think and your manager should genuinely listen, consider and respond to your views.

TAKE IMMEDIATE ACTION

Don't always blame others if you were left out from a decision-making process; you have to shoulder some of the responsibility. Ask yourself why you were not included. Don't get angry, don't procrastinate and don't bottle it up. Go and speak to your manager before you speak to anyone else. Remain calm and ask why you were not consulted. They may have simply forgotten.

If you have views or alternative solutions, then let them know. If you feel there will be serious consequences which may not have been considered, make these very clear. Follow up your discussion with an e-mail confirming what you discussed. You can address the e-mail to any others involved in the decision-making process, so that they may also consider your views, but if you do, you should consider your wording very carefully. Avoid giving the impression that you are being disloyal to your manager. Ultimately you may not be able to change the decision made, but it helps if your views are made clear and considered.

PREVENT IT HAPPENING AGAIN

Treat this as a learning experience, and take action to reduce the risk of it happening again. If you find that your manager genuinely forgot to include you or did not realise the importance of involving you, then it is clear that you have not been making enough effort to communicate with them on a regular basis. Make sure you do so in future.

Don't just contact your manager when you have a problem or when they call a meeting. Make the effort to see your line manager regularly to update them on current issues. Keep them informed of everything you are doing. It is also important to keep them up-to-date with any projects or work that have been delegated to you.

Nurses are generally not good at promoting themselves, but if you do not promote your knowledge and expertise, how else is your manager going to know? It is not sufficient to say that it's their job to find out. It's also your job to let them know and get yourself involved in activities, meetings and projects in which your knowledge and expertise are required.

ORGANISATION-WIDE DECISIONS

If senior management (e.g. the chief executive or board of directors) within your organisation make a decision which affects you and your team detrimentally and you were not consulted, you do have the right to make a written request for information and consultation, under the Information and Consultation of Employees Regulations (Department of Trade and Industry 2006). However, 10% of the rest of the workforce must also want this information. To make use of this or any legislation, you should always consult with human resources (HR) and your union representative in the first instance.

IS IT BULLYING?

If you feel you are doing everything you can to improve communications with your manager but feel that you are being deliberately left out of decision making, this could be construed as bullying. It is advisable in this situation that you keep file notes. Record all incidents where you have not been consulted and note all actions you have taken to try to improve the situation.

Try and speak to your manager first. Tell them how their actions are making you feel. Discuss your concerns and agree actions to be taken in the future. If your manager refuses to change or even to listen to you, seek further advice from a senior HR advisor. They will guide you through the process outlined in your local policy for bullying and harassment. They will also provide you with support and access to counselling if required.

ACT, IF A CHANGE IN ANOTHER DEPARTMENT HAS A KNOCK-ON EFFECT IN YOURS

Health care is continually changing to meet differing demands, with performance indicators and financial restrictions complicating the process. We barely have a chance to settle down after one move, merger or restructuring of services when the next change is being announced. Decisions may have to be made quickly, and sometimes they are not properly thought through. Certain aspects can be overlooked, particularly the effects on neighbouring departments.

Mistakes happen. Don't put up with the consequences and just make the best of things. A common example is disruption through building work. The facilities department may be doing building work nearby and you find the noise is intolerable for patients returning from theatre who need optimum rest to recover. Don't just moan about the system and accept it. Nurses are so good at coping with severe disruptions that often they will think nothing of it. But you must not continue to cope if it is affecting the patients. You are the patients' advocate and it is your duty to ensure that patients do not suffer unduly.

Shouting at a member of the facilities department over the telephone will probably have little effect either. Gather your information or data first. Find out:

- Who else is affected?
- Are they suffering in silence too?
- What has anyone else tried to do about it?
- Who is the senior person in charge of the project?
- Was your line manager(s) involved or consulted?

It is sometimes the case that the manager was consulted and gave permission for the work to go ahead but forgot to inform everyone concerned or did not realise the impact of the decision on the wards. If this is the case, contacting the manager of the facilities department first is not appropriate. Your manager should be the first person to contact.

Don't just complain to your line manager and expect them to resolve the issue (even if they are partly to blame). That is commonly known as 'passing the buck' and is not always appropriate. State the problem and work together on possible solutions. Present your case together to the appropriate manager of the building works project, preferably face-to-face, and follow up your discussion and agreed actions with an e-mail. Keep your line manager informed and involved at each stage in the process.

Remember to always keep records and copies of e-mails. Suggest solutions once you have all the facts, such as cancelling surgery, closing beds and transferring patients to other wards temporarily. Work with the facilities manager and your own line manager in finding suitable solutions. Don't focus on the fact that you were not consulted in the planning process.

COPING IS NOT TAKING ACTION

Another common example of poorly considered change concerns decisions regarding bed management. Sometimes, the specialty of some beds or even whole wards is changed at short notice. As many nurses and nurse managers are aware, these sorts of decisions can be catastrophic for patients, but non-clinical managers are not always aware of the full implications. Don't just cope. Coping in situations like these could be tantamount to negligence.

If this happens to you, it is advisable to:

- make a full risk assessment, including getting your team to identify all the potential issues and problems
- make an appointment to discuss the issue with your line manager, general manager and the bed manager together, and agree alternative solutions for the benefit of the patients. This could include delaying the start date to ensure your team are appropriately trained through secondments to other wards and specialist courses
- document the outcomes of the discussion and circulate to the appropriate people.

In summary, if you find someone makes a decision that has huge 'knock-on' effects in your department without consulting you, take appropriate action. Coping is not taking action.

DON'T BE PRESSURISED INTO TAKING ON EXTRA WORK WITHOUT FUNDING

With budgetary problems commonplace, being pressured to take on extra work is a common problem within health care. Because patient care might be compromised, health care professionals often feel they have no choice but to take on the extra work. Unfortunately, nurses are often too willing to regularly go without breaks, work double shifts, stay on regularly at the end of shifts for a couple of hours (unpaid) and take work home so that patients will not suffer. It is not a fair situation. Some managers may pressurise you into taking on extra work; others may take on the extra work and expect you to follow suit. You should not allow yourself to be cajoled into accepting more and more work without appropriate funding.

EMERGENCY SITUATIONS

In emergency situations, you have no choice. If you have to take a number of patients who require additional care and need to book extra agency staff, then so be it. But make it clear in such situations that you do not have the funds within your budget to deal with these extra demands. Work out afterwards, with the help of your finance advisor, roughly what the cost will be and inform your line manager. Make sure your discussion is documented and a copy sent to your line manager and whoever else is involved in making the decision: that includes members of your hospital board if necessary.

NON-EMERGENCY SITUATIONS

If you are asked or 'told' to take on extra work (such as taking patients from a different specialty), arrange a meeting with both your line manager and finance advisor to clarify and agree how much the extra work will cost. Do this even if your manager has told you not to worry about it and that they will 'sort it out'. These situations do not always get 'sorted out'. You need to make sure that everyone is clear about how much you will be over-spent at the end of year as a result.

If your line manager informs you that they will or have accessed funding from elsewhere for the extra work, get this in writing first. It does not have to be formal; an e-mail will suffice.

OPENING UP EXTRA BEDS

If you open up extra beds, make sure you have the appropriate staff to provide an acceptable level of patient care. Don't cope with your existing staffing levels if it is unsafe or reduces the standard of care. If you do, you are indicating that you do not need extra staff for those beds. How can you prove that this work needs extra funding when you appear to have coped well without it? It is not unknown for some ward managers who were asked to open up some extra beds temporarily to deal with a short-term problem to find themselves a few years down the line with those beds having remained open but still with the original funded staffing establishment. Don't let it happen to you.

PROJECT WORK

If you are asked to take on a piece of work on behalf of the directorate or the organisation, such as an audit, clarify how much time and resources it will take (remember that staff time is a resource). If you are required to undertake the work personally, identify and agree with your manager which aspect of your existing workload you will not do, in order to make time to do this extra work. Even a piece of work such as investigating a complaint or incident for another area could take a few days or weeks.

If members of your team are required to do extra work such as new link nurse roles or attending organisation-wide working groups, calculate how many hours' work will be required and work out how much that will cost you in terms of clinical cover. Don't expect staff to take the work home or, worse still, to leave their patients with an unacceptable standard of supervision/care in order to undertake the extra work required with these roles.

If a member of staff needs to take on a new link nurse role, for example, work out how much time they will need to fulfil the role. It may need the link nurse to:

- attend a 2-hour meeting each month
- take follow-up actions from each meeting
- keep the ward team informed and up-to-date regularly
- deliver teaching sessions.

The above tasks may require the equivalent of 1–2 days' worth of additional work per month. How much will this cost in terms of agency cover? Even if you find the link nurse stays on for a short time after each shift to fulfil the duties required and accrues time owed, the time they eventually take will come out of your budget. It costs money to cover a shift or half a shift when the nurse takes her time back. There is no allowance within your funded establishment to cover 'time owed' (see Ch. 6).

WORK WITH YOUR MANAGER

If you regularly say yes to more work, your manager will probably assume you have the time and the resources to do it. Some do not realise the impact of such decisions in terms of your workload. It's up to you make it clear what impact the extra work will have.

However, it is not wise to refuse *all* extra work completely because you have no funding. Just make sure that you:

● clarify the cost and implications of the extra work
● discuss alternative solutions
● agree terms and conditions in writing with your line manager.

IF YOU ARE DOING EXTRA WORK WITHOUT FUNDING, TAKE ACTION

If you have taken on extra work such as extra beds, with the promise of funding that somehow never arrived, you will probably be over-spent on your budget. Your priority now is to make sure that you are not labelled as the ward manager who is unable to manage their budget. Work out exactly how much the extra work is costing you in terms of staff time and supplies. Do this together with your finance advisor. Continually remind your manager(s) of the sum of money over and above your budget that you are spending on this extra work.

If you are working within your budget, then you have proved that you do not need extra staff and resources in order to have these extra beds. No manager will be provided with extra funding through the yearly business planning process for a team that is completing the required work within their given budget.

If you are expected to continue with the extra work without extra funding, you have two choices:

1. Get it in writing that your manager agrees you may go over budget by a set amount in order to deliver the extra work or staff the extra beds.
2. Work out with your team which aspects of work need to be sacrificed in order to keep within budget, as well as ensuring the patients are safe and well cared for. Agree your actions in writing with your manager. If your manager does not agree, you must come up with alternative actions.

If you do not do either of the above, you are effectively sanctioning the compromising of health and safety standards on your ward. You would be allowing your staff to cope with increased workloads and paving the way for mistakes to be made. You could therefore be taking responsibility for the consequences of someone else's decision. Beware of being made a scapegoat.

KEEP THE COMMUNICATION CHANNELS OPEN

Do not wait until you are asked about what is going on in your ward; keep your manager informed. If your line manager's office is in a different building or even on a different site, do not use this as an excuse. Blaming others for your predicament is a reactive approach and indicative of poor leadership. Use e-mail to keep your manager up-to-date with events. It's up to you to build up the relationship to ensure you have the right support and contacts for the good of your ward and your team.

Even if your line manager shows little interest in your ward or department, make sure you still keep regular contact and let them know what is happening. Leave out details that are not their concern, e.g. dealing with minor staff mistakes or problems with the roster. Give them a general overview of the themes of complaints, incidents and staffing issues. Remember also to highlight any achievements.

WHY SOME MANAGERS 'MICROMANAGE'

When you go to your manager with any concerns, try to present some potential solutions rather than dwell on the problems. If you always expect your manager to come up with the solutions and sort out your problems, you are at risk of being 'micromanaged'. This situation occurs when line managers begin to get too involved in the details of management at ward level, such as personnel problems or roster issues, and may even hold meetings with members of your team. This sort of behaviour can indicate that your manager does not have confidence in your abilities to manage your unit.

If this is happening to you, try to focus on your own behaviour before changing theirs. Think through and find out what you could do to resolve each individual problem that occurs, before seeing your manager. Phone the relevant 'expert' (e.g. HR advisor, finance advisor, bed manager) to find out the appropriate information you need and perhaps discuss possible options first. If, for example, a member of your staff comes to you complaining that they are being bullied, and you are not sure what steps to take, don't go immediately to your line manager. Call your HR advisor first for advice about the options you can take within the policy for bullying and harassment. Ask your colleagues (other ward managers) if they have had similar experiences that you could learn from. Once you have all the information, then go to your line manager and either:

- let them know what course of action you have decided to take, or
- present the options you have found for resolving the problem and ask for their opinion on the matter.

Show your manager that you have initiative. Don't burden them with even more problems on top of their own workload.

KEEP IN CONSTANT CONTACT

As you gain more experience over the years, you will need less support from your manager. On the other hand, try not to fall into the trap of getting on with things so well that they don't bother with you and what is happening on your ward. Contact them regularly, at least once a week, and give them a general update. This will ensure they are aware of the good practice on your ward and will remember to keep you involved in wider issues.

If you have any untoward incidents, let your manager know not only about the remedial action that has been taken but also what you are going to do to reduce the risk of it happening again. This prevents more senior managers telling you to change aspects of care on your ward as a result of receiving incident forms. It is better for you and your team to identify and implement the necessary changes first, before being told to.

GIVE FEEDBACK

It is a good idea to give your line manager regular feedback just as you do with your team. You want to be able to encourage all the positive aspects of their behaviour and make them aware of aspects which have a negative effect. If your manager comes to see you regularly each week and you appreciate that, say so. If your manager has a tendency to interfere unnecessarily with the work of your team, your frustration may not be understood unless you say so. In this case, the manager may think they are helping you and could have no idea unless you maintain an open and honest dialogue.

Similarly, try to encourage some feedback from your manager so that you have some idea how you are progressing. Some managers may not give feedback unless asked.

WRITE CLEAR AND TIMELY REPORTS

Getting reports finished on time and done properly will help enormously in building a good relationship with your manager. Try not to put all report-writing tasks to the bottom of your in-tray. Start the process immediately. It prevents you spending precious time worrying about when you are going to get the time to do it. Developing a basic outline to start with should help you to be clearer in your mind about what information is required and you may even be able to delegate parts of the report where appropriate.

When asked by your line manager to write a report, it is advisable to confirm the objective of the report and who the reader(s) will be before you start work on it. Taking time to check this at the beginning can save you hours of wasted effort later on. It should help you to decide what information to include or leave out, and hopefully prevent your manager saying after all your hard work, 'This is not what I asked for'.

STAGE 1: WRITE A BASIC OUTLINE

Write a basic outline before you start researching or investigating the information that you will need. It will help direct your investigation. All reports should be based on the following headings, which can be individually adapted at a later stage:

1. Executive summary (and recommendations if any).
2. Introduction (based on the objective).
3. Background (include the method of investigation/research).

4. Results (and any implementation).
5. Conclusion.

Start any report with these five basic headings to guide you. It prevents you from sitting down and staring at a piece of blank paper wondering where to begin.

STAGE 2: THE INTRODUCTION

The introduction is one of the most important sections of a report. The reader can form an opinion about the rest of the report based on the clarity and quality of the introduction. It's a good idea to use the objective you have agreed with your manager to form the basis of the introduction to your report.

STAGE 3: BACKGROUND DESCRIPTION

Describe the background to the report, i.e. make the context clear. Keep it in note form in the initial stages to stop you becoming too focused on this section. If your report is about how you have done something to come up with a solution, use this section to describe the process you used. It is often better to complete this section once you have finished the rest of the report.

STAGE 4: RESULTS/IMPLEMENTATION

This is the main part of the report. A good idea to get started is to list everything you want to include in the report then group points into key headings. You could write down each item on a 'post-it' note then sort the 'post-it' notes into general themes or key headings. Once you have done this you can concentrate on researching or finding the information to put in under each heading, and delegating some parts to your team or others if appropriate.

STAGE 5: CONCLUSION AND RECOMMENDATIONS

Use this section to conclude the main findings or recommendations.

STAGE 6: EXECUTIVE SUMMARY

It's easier to write this after writing the report, although it needs to be inserted at the beginning. It should be a brief summary of the report with any recommendations. This should enable the reader to get an overview of what is in the report without having to read it through.

Further tips

When you come to the writing part, there are a few rules to remember:

1. Write in the first person, 'I'; not 'one' or 'the author'.
2. Don't use jargon such as 'obs' or 'resps'.
3. Use active, not passive phrases (e.g. 'we decided' rather than 'it was decided').

4. Avoid exclamation marks.
5. Try to avoid using superfluous phrases such as 'at this moment in time' instead of 'now', or 'in respect of' instead of 'about'.
6. Paragraphs should be wider than they are long.
7. Explain all abbreviations, keeping in mind that some people who read the report will not be health care professionals.
8. Ensure the report has page numbers.

As a general rule, any reports should be short and succinct and include more facts than descriptions. Few managers will read long reports from cover to cover. Most will read the introduction, key headings, conclusion and recommendations, so concentrate on those aspects.

Always give reports in on time. Remember to under-promise and over-deliver. If you think it will take you 2 weeks, set a time limit of 3–4 weeks and aim to give it in at 2 weeks. Managers are usually impressed by people who deliver work early or on time.

KNOW HOW TO CONDUCT A GOOD INVESTIGATION

You may be asked by your line manager to undertake a full investigation into matters involving issues such as:

● allegations of bullying or harassment
● poor performance or misconduct
● allegations of criminal activity, negligence or deliberate harm.

Usually you would not undertake a formal investigation into staff behaviour on your own ward. It is good practice to appoint investigators who are not involved in the incident or line manage the area in which the involved member(s) of staff work. (Remember that complaint and incident investigations are not formal and therefore require a different informal investigation which is usually carried out by you and your team in your own area.)

Before commencing any formal investigation, confirm the following with your manager:

1. Exactly what is to be investigated and under which policy.
2. The time frame for completion. You will need to negotiate dedicated time in which to carry out the investigation. Do not attempt to do this in your own time, or in quiet times during your shift. You will require cover for your time out.
3. Who you can go to for support. You should have access to an experienced HR advisor throughout the process.

MAKE A PROVISIONAL PLAN OF ACTION

Agree a plan of action with your manager. This plan may change as new information comes to light but you should start off with a plan so you can estimate the time it will take.

Your first step in your plan is usually to arrange the interview dates. It takes considerable time to arrange venues, dates and times. Do not carry out the interviews until you have reviewed all the necessary documentary evidence, but try and do them as quickly as possible after the event in order to:

- ensure the event(s) is still fresh in everyone's mind
- stop rumours and gossip
- reduce unnecessary anxiety for all those involved
- reduce unnecessary waste of resources if anyone has been suspended.

When you arrange the interviews, you must ensure that each person is informed of their right to have a trade union representative or work colleague to accompany them. It is up to them to arrange this. You should also let them know of any support that your organisation offers such as trained counsellors for victims of alleged bullying. You should ensure that the alleged wrong-doer is informed of the investigation as soon as possible. It would be unfair for the witnesses or anyone else to hear of the investigation before them. You should also keep the ward/department manager informed as well as your own line manager.

REVIEW ALL THE DOCUMENTARY EVIDENCE

It's advisable to make photocopies of any documentary evidence to prevent tampering of records. Keep a record of all documents reviewed as part of the process. Relevant documents may include:

- rosters
- ward induction/development programmes
- patients' medical or nursing records
- local policies/guidelines
- any relevant professional or national guidelines.

Remember to follow the confidentiality guidelines if any patient information is required for the investigation (see p. 124).

INTERVIEWS

Interviews usually start with the person who raised the issue. This is to establish the nature of the complaint or allegation and any further information which may be relevant. You will also need to interview the alleged wrong-doer(s) to give them the chance to put across their version of events. Any witnesses will need to be interviewed as well as the line manager. If you are investigating a matter of which you have no knowledge or experience, you may also need to interview other professionals for their expert advice. Witnesses are usually entitled to time off in lieu or payment if interviewed outside of normal working hours. Check your organisational policy and inform their line managers of the time required if this is the case.

Before you start an interview, you should prepare your questions to ensure you cover all the required areas. At the beginning of the interview, take time to do the following:

1. Make the person feel comfortable with appropriate refreshments and seating.
2. Reiterate their right to be accompanied by a trade union representative or work colleague.
3. Explain that this is not disciplinary action and that your role is only to establish the facts.
4. Explain that they should not discuss the case with anyone else who is involved.

Keep a record of all the interviews. Give each person the opportunity to read through the notes of their interview and sign that they agree it is an accurate reflection of what was discussed. They may prefer to provide their own statements. Make sure they are aware that any statements may be used as evidence in the event of a subsequent disciplinary hearing.

Don't be concerned about calling people back to re-interview. You may find you have to do this as further information comes to light. Remember that all information obtained should remain confidential so do not share information about anyone else's interview with subsequent interviewees. In practice, this can be quite difficult to achieve so be vigilant.

PREPARE A WRITTEN REPORT

The following headings can be used as a general guide, but check your organisation's policy for local guidance on what is expected within your report:

● Executive summary (no more than 10 lines).
● Introduction – include terms of reference or objective.
● Description of the issue and/or allegations and an outline of the investigative process including timetable of interviews.
● Findings – list them clearly. You may wish to list them under headings of each complaint. Refer to witnesses either by their initials or as witness A, B or C, etc. throughout the report.
● Conclusions – is the complaint or allegation substantiated?
● Recommendations.
● Appendices.

The purpose of an investigation is to establish the facts. It does not equate to disciplinary action. It may or may not lead to a disciplinary hearing. If it does, the evidence provided in the investigative report will help inform the disciplinary panel.

ACTION POINTS

- If you haven't already had one within the past year, make an appointment with your manager for an appraisal and ensure your objectives are congruent with theirs.
- Arrange regular meetings with your manager throughout the rest of the year to review your set objectives and to keep them informed of progress on your ward.
- If your manager leaves you out of decision making or any changes, make a point of trying to improve your working relationship with them to reduce the risk of it happening again.
- If a change takes place that is detrimental to patient care, gather the facts and approach the appropriate people with the support of your manager.
- Try not to present any problems to your manager; present solutions or options for action each time.
- Always calculate the monetary costs for any extra work, whether or not funding has been granted.
- Give regular feedback to your manager, particularly with a job done well. Invite lots of feedback from your manager to ensure you are continually improving your own performance.
- Take on the delegation of an investigation as a challenge and opportune learning experience.
- Always start reports early and give them in early or on time.

Reference

Department of Trade and Industry, 2006. The Information and Consultation of Employees Regulations: DTI guidance. Online. Available: http://www.bis.gov.uk/files/file25934.pdf Feb 2012.

MANAGE DIFFICULT SITUATIONS

Managers have to deal with all sorts of different personalities ranging from the shy and passive to the explosive and aggressive types. Working in the health care environment can bring out the worst in people as the pressure increases with more work and fewer resources. It is important to understand the emotional vulnerability that underlies many difficult situations. A key managerial skill is the ability to notice individual needs for recognition and self-esteem, and to be confident in confronting challenging situations and people in a constructive and positive manner.

THE DIFFICULT MANAGER

People usually get promoted because they are good at their job. The problem with clinicians being good at their job is that when promoted to become managers, they find it is a totally different job from that which they were doing before. They do not necessarily have the skills in managing people or resources. (In some cases, people are promoted because they are poor clinicians or because they have been in the organisation for a very long time, but this is rare nowadays.) That's not to say that all managers are no good because most are (even those who may not have been appropriate for the job originally). Many will thrive and become good managers in time. Unfortunately, there are a few who do not. Some will struggle in their role and may take out their frustrations on others or perhaps become very controlling and manipulative. Some adopt an aggressive manner and may shout or lose their temper on occasions, while others may shy away from difficult decisions and leave their team to their own devices.

MANAGERS WHO ARE PRONE TO GETTING ANGRY

If your manager starts shouting at you, do not sit and take it but, whatever you do, do not shout back. Say that you are sorry about whatever it is, but would rather wait and discuss the matter when things have calmed down. Say that you will leave if necessary. Only stay if they agree to talk to you in a civil manner. By saying that you prefer to wait until things have calmed down, it does not look like you are blaming them. You need to be diplomatic. After all, this is your manager.

Unfortunately there are some managers who are continuously aggressive and intimidating. Explain that this approach of shouting at you is not going to make you work any harder. It just serves to upset and intimidate you. If you have made a mistake, always admit to it. If you have not done something that was asked for, state clearly and succinctly the reasons why you have not achieved what is required. Don't make excuses, which may only serve to increase their anger.

If this is a situation that comes up time and time again, go and discuss it through with either your manager's line manager or someone senior in your human resources (HR) department. It's best to let your manager know first of your intentions. This may well stop the situation by itself. All NHS organisations are required to have a policy for dealing with bullying and harassment. You should be well supported through the process (although you must keep a factual log of all incidents as evidence).

MANAGERS WHO DON'T MANAGE

Some managers are reluctant to take on their managerial responsibilities. These tend to be people who are promoted because of their clinical experience. As mentioned previously, clinical skills are not the same as managerial skills.

These types of managers may busy themselves with issues that require their clinical expertise and ignore their managerial role. It can be hard to get them to make any decisions or take any action on important managerial matters.

It is difficult to deal with this sort of manager because they are normally well liked and maintain a good rapport with everyone. They will spend a lot of time sympathising with you and your team over your issues, but don't actually do anything about them. People tend to label them as 'supportive' managers because they spend time listening to individual problems (despite not doing anything about them).

One way of dealing with this type of manager is to never present issues as problems, try and present the full solution to the problem, or a number of alternative solutions from which the manager can choose. For each solution, make sure:

- it has been fully researched and meets the appropriate guidelines or policy
- the appropriate people have been consulted
- the implications have been considered in depth.

Bear in mind that these managers tend to thrive on social acceptance among the clinical team so ensure you make it clear that your solutions have been generated by your team and reflect all their views too.

MANAGERS WHO EXPECT TOO MUCH

It is hard for managers whose working day used to revolve around patients' needs to enter a world where it revolves around managing others from an office environment. Patients' needs were always the priority, but when the next role no longer entails looking after patients, it can be difficult to work out what the priorities are. Some will take on too much work in order to compensate for this and over the years may get into a pattern of being very busy but not actually achieving anything. Some will take on extra projects or find it difficult to say no when bombarded with demands from their own senior managers, especially with regard to meeting the latest 'performance indicator'.

The problem for you is that some managers end up working extra long hours (unpaid of course) and expect you to do the same. You may find that some of this extra work is being delegated down to you. If this is happening to you and it gets too much (and you are certain that you are managing your own time effectively) then you must say so. Work out what your priorities and time commitments are (see Ch. 2) then go and discuss them with your manager. This can achieve two things:

1. Your manager will hopefully stop delegating the extra work to you.
2. Having seen what you have done, your manager may be stimulated into defining and prioritising their own workload using the same formula.

THE PROBLEMATIC COLLEAGUE

The very nature of our work means we will always be working with people, sometimes some very difficult people. Unfortunately you cannot choose your work colleagues, and in the clinically focused role of the ward manager, you cannot retreat to an office or work alone to avoid the problem.

So how do you handle a colleague who is proving rather difficult to work with? First, tell them. This sounds fairly obvious but you would be amazed at how many don't do this. The individual then carries on blissfully unaware of the angst they are causing. The situation will get worse if you leave it, and the longer you leave telling your colleague, the worse they will feel. Second, don't get personal, otherwise they will become defensive and you'll get nowhere. Focus on the issue, not the person.

COLLEAGUES WHO TEND TO BE CONTINUALLY NEGATIVE

Negative people are those who tend to be insecure and unsure of themselves. By saying negative things about others they are often trying to cover up their own limitations. Make an effort to share your ideas with them. Get them on your side by offering to take on some work together. Boost their confidence by giving them positive feedback on things they do well.

COLLEAGUES WHO CONTINUALLY WHINGE ABOUT OTHERS

If you have a colleague who is always finding fault with people, ask what they have done or plan to do about the problem:

● 'What have you done about his behaviour?'
● 'Have you told her how you feel?'

The more often you question what they have done about it, the less they will find fault.

COLLEAGUES WHO PUT THEMSELVES DOWN ALL THE TIME

Colleagues who turn the criticism on themselves, saying things like 'I'm not good enough', are usually lacking in confidence. It's easier to criticise themselves before anyone else does. With a colleague like this, you can help simply by telling them that they are doing a good job and to stop talking themselves down. Those who put themselves down in order to receive compliments and praise from others are equally annoying. You have to be blunt in this case and say something like 'Look, you know how good you are at that sort of thing and hardly need any more feedback from me to boost your confidence'.

COLLEAGUES WHO ARE CONTINUALLY CALLING FOR ADVICE AND SUPPORT

Some of your less experienced colleagues may have found you so helpful in the past that they continue to turn to you for every problem they encounter. If this happens, encourage them to seek a mentor/clinical supervisor for extra support. Tell them that relying on you alone for advice and guidance will restrict their learning; they have to seek support from others as well as you. Don't do things for them or you will encourage the behaviour. Whenever this person calls you, always ask them first what they think is the best action and enable them to come to their own conclusions and actions.

ALLEGATIONS OF BULLYING OR HARASSMENT WITHIN YOUR TEAM

WHAT IS BULLYING OR HARASSMENT?

If members of your team do not treat their colleagues with dignity and respect, it could be interpreted as bullying or harassment. Situations in which a member of your team feels threatened, insulted or intimidated in any way by another person's behaviour must be stopped immediately. If any of your staff come to you saying that someone else makes them feel this way, even if it was not intended, you need to take action. If you don't do anything:

1. The individual's confidence and self-esteem will plummet and therefore affect their standard of work.
2. Other staff will get involved and begin to take sides, thus creating tension within the team.

You should take all complaints seriously, even if you personally believe that it is simply a case of firm management or a harmless joke. Bullying and harassment are defined as any sort of behaviour which makes an individual feel upset, threatened, humiliated or vulnerable and undermines their confidence. In other words, it is the *impact* of the behaviour, not the *intent* of the perpetrator which determines whether the person is being bullied or harassed.

Be aware that bullying can include:

- regular shouting or criticism in front of others
- refusing to speak to someone directly
- excessive supervision or checking up on a colleague's work
- constantly giving menial or trivial tasks to others
- deliberately excluding individuals from work-related social events
- unreasonably refusing requests for time off or training.

Harassment is any unwanted behaviour towards an individual regarding gender, race, disability, sexual orientation, religion, beliefs or any personal characteristic. This can include:

- intrusive questioning or gossiping about a person's private life, religion, activities, sexual orientation, etc.
- being condescending about the way a person dresses or speaks
- insensitive jokes or pranks
- unnecessary body contact.

WHAT STEPS SHOULD YOU TAKE?

When a member of staff complains to you that another person's behaviour is insulting or demeaning, your first step is to encourage them to tell the perpetrator, if they have not already done so. Sometimes people do not realise the effect they are having on others. Once informed, many will alter their behaviour.

The individual who came to you may be low in confidence and therefore may need your support to do this. It is far better to work through with the individual what approach to take and encourage them to do it for themselves. This will increase their self-esteem and enable them to deal with any future situations with more confidence. However, the situation may be such that you will need to act as mediator between the two parties. In this case, make sure you have both parties present, otherwise you will get caught between two different versions of events and not know who to believe.

WHAT DO YOU DO IF YOUR INITIAL APPROACH DOES NOT WORK?

If the perpetrator does not change their behaviour, you may have to intervene and use a more direct approach. In other words, tell the perpetrator to change their behaviour. If this does not work, the staff member at this stage can take a more formal approach by putting their concerns in writing. You should be liaising closely with your HR advisor throughout the process and ensuring that both parties involved in the allegation have access to support from their trade union representatives.

Once a formal allegation is made, a manager from outside your ward will usually be brought in to undertake a formal investigation. This means that those involved, including you and other staff members, will be interviewed and statements taken. A report will be written with recommendations as to what actions should be taken. The recommended actions could include a number of things such as:

- an apology
- transfer of either party to another ward or department
- counselling or time off
- identification of training needs
- a disciplinary hearing.

Every NHS organisation is required to have a specific policy and guidelines for cases of bullying and harassment. It is wise to make yourself familiar with this policy. Also ensure your team are familiar with what your organisation defines as bullying and harassment. It will increase their awareness that bullying and harassment do not just concern people who shout and use violent threatening behaviour.

STAFF COMPLAINTS

Hopefully, you will have created a good healthy working atmosphere so that your team will be happy to bring issues to your attention if they have any concerns about their working conditions, standards of patient care or relationships with colleagues. Your leadership style should also ensure that all staff are willing to work together to agree some sort of solution. This includes taking the time to listen to their concerns and being willing to help them work through the issue and ensure something is done to resolve the situation.

COMPLAINTS IN WRITING

If people think of you as not particularly approachable or if any staff members are unhappy with your response to their concerns, they can raise a formal grievance. A grievance is basically a written complaint from a member of staff. If a member of staff has to write a formal letter to you or your manager to make a complaint, you should seriously question your approach as a manager. Generally, staff will only resort to this after they have exhausted all other options, which mainly consists of getting you to listen to them and take note of their concerns.

All NHS organisations are required to have a grievance procedure, and it is usually very strict in terms of the timetable to which you have to keep. If you receive a written complaint from a member of your staff about their working conditions, standards of care or relationships with colleagues, you should invite them to meet with you as soon as possible and inform them that they have a right to be accompanied by a friend, colleague or trade union representative. If the solution is outside your authority or if the grievance is against you personally, you should refer the matter to your line manager.

Most policies state that you must have a meeting with them within a certain number of days from receipt of the letter; always check your local policy as it is normally a very short time span.

At this meeting you should:

1. Allow the staff member to explain their complaint and what they think the solution should be.
2. Discuss and agree a solution, or if you are not sure what to do about the complaint, you can then adjourn the meeting while you seek further advice.
3. Follow up the meeting with a letter confirming what was agreed. Your policy will state when this is to be done. It is usually within 3–5 days following the meeting.

WHAT TO DO IF YOU CANNOT RESOLVE THE COMPLAINT ALONE

If the complaint is not resolved, the individual can write to your line manager who, in turn, can either meet with them to discuss the issue or send a written response. Again, your policy will set a time limit for the response, which is usually within 3–5 days from receipt of the letter.

If your line manager cannot resolve the issue, the individual can then take it to the next managerial level. Again, they will either meet with the individual or write a letter. If the individual is still not satisfied, they can raise an appeal at board level.

At this stage, one of the board directors will arrange an appeal panel. They will consider all the evidence including statements from any witnesses or representatives. The appeal panel decision is final.

HELPING YOUR STAFF TO ACT

You may be personally confident in dealing with difficult people when you are on duty but part of your role is to make sure that your team are equipped with the skills to deal with difficult people and situations when you are not there.

THE ARROGANT CONSULTANT

Working partnerships between medical and nursing staff have not always been easy. The differences in pay, status, education and gender have historically led to a clash in perspectives and tensions in the working environment. Nowadays, on balance, things have changed for the better. Nursing training is more academically focused than in the past and nursing roles and responsibilities have expanded to include many of those previously done by junior doctors. The nursing profession nowadays is less hierarchical and more patient centred. However, the medical profession generally remains fairly rigid in its career structure, with the junior doctors doing all the running around and the consultants being the bosses who give the orders. There are some consultants who still feel they are the ultimate boss and everyone should do as they say and 'woe betide' those who dare to question their decisions. These types are rare but still around, and can be quite difficult to handle.

Sometimes the arrogance is a cover-up for the fact that they do have a highly stressful job and may well suffer from inner feelings of inadequacy. How many times have you given a consultant any positive feedback on their work, or seen others do so? It can be quite an isolating role, especially for those who have had no training and development in communication or leadership skills. How do they know what they need? They have only recently got used to the idea of having formal appraisals.

One way of dealing with this behaviour is to put extra effort into building up a good working relationship with them right from the start. Give positive feedback regularly and any negative feedback will be taken more seriously. It you only give negative feedback (i.e. keep telling them that their behaviour is unacceptable on your ward), they will assume that you are simply whingeing all the time. You will be seen as the problem, not them.

Do not encourage your staff to confront them about their behaviour. Few will acknowledge that they are arrogant and can be very patronising and hurtful, particularly if some of your staff are shy or less confident in themselves. Instead, show your staff how to talk to all consultants with confidence and how to give regular feedback. Include your staff in all areas of decision making including ward rounds. Always encourage them to join in any discussions with your support rather than to be passive bystanders.

THE PUSHY BED MANAGER

Bed managers can never please everyone. A&E staff get fed up with them because patients are stacking up, ward staff are fed up with them for constantly pestering about the 'bed state' and discharges, managers are constantly pestering them to meet the contract numbers; they get hassled from all sides. It's no wonder that they may pressurise your staff to discharge too early or to admit patients when they are not ready.

When you are on duty, it shouldn't be a problem. But what do you do if your staff are coerced into making decisions when you are not there; decisions that may not be appropriate such as taking extra or inappropriate patients into an already overstretched team of staff? It is difficult to refuse, especially if a matron or general manager becomes involved. If you find this has happened when you return from 'days off', the first thing to do is to speak to the bed manager as soon as you can to ascertain the facts. It's not unusual for staff to exaggerate a little when in reality they did little to explain their position to the bed manager.

If you find out that members of your staff were forced into compromising patient care in order to meet targets, then explain to the bed manager that you are not happy and will not allow it to happen again in the future. Confirm the discussion plus your agreed actions briefly by e-mail. Keep a file note of the conversation. This is usually enough to ensure it does not happen again. If it does happen again, do the same and involve more senior managers if necessary. The appropriate people must be made aware of what is happening.

In the meantime, make sure that you set criteria with your team about bed decisions such as when to declare a bed is ready to take the next patient, i.e. when the patient is no longer on the ward, or can wait in the dayroom only if they are fit and do not require any nursing care or attention while there. Make sure the bed manager, matron and general manager are fully aware and involved in the development of these guidelines. Your organisation may already have some, so don't write new ones unless your ward or department is an exception.

OVERLOADED LINK NURSES

Always be aware about what your link nurses are being asked to do. Their role is to act as a link between the nurse specialist or practice development team and the wards. These nurse specialists and practice development teams usually have a huge agenda and have targets to implement across the organisation. Often the only way they can communicate is through the link nurses. It is an effective system of disseminating information. Unfortunately, some will use the nurses to do their work for them. Your nurses may not realise that they are being used to fulfil the objectives of others.

Junior staff in particular may be eager to please and do the required work in their own time. Their dedication to improving patient care can be abused. Don't allow this to happen to your staff. Make sure you are fully aware of the demands placed upon them, and intervene if necessary. Give them permission to say no. They should be doing work which benefits the team and patient care on your ward, not the person who is leading the link nurses.

DEALING WITH RACISM OR OTHER FORMS OF DISCRIMINATION

PATIENTS AND RELATIVES

If a patient or relative refuses care because they object to the nurse's appearance, skin colour, religion, etc., despite the fact that the person is a competent nurse, then it should not be tolerated. This sounds simple but there are still recent examples in which health care professionals were not supported by their managers when discriminated against by patients or relatives. In 2004, a nurse was awarded £20 000 in compensation when a relative asked that she not look after her baby because she was black. The manager moved the baby to another ward. In 2006, a male nurse won a case of sex discrimination because he was not allowed to undertake procedures in his training such as ECGs on female patients without a chaperone.

If patients or relatives on your ward discriminate against your staff in any way, make sure you support them by telling the patient or relative that their comments are offensive. Remain polite and respectful. You will not be able to change the person's views, so it is not wise to attempt it. Just explain that their behaviour will not be tolerated. All members of your team should be assured that they will have your full support in any cases of this kind. Never dismiss any discriminatory comments as trivial and do not move the patient or nurse unless the nurse specifically requests not to look after them. If the patient or relative refuses care on discriminatory grounds, they should be made aware that they are effectively refusing services altogether.

If the patient or relative will not listen to you or the nurse involved, consult your organisation's zero tolerance policy. All NHS organisations are required to have such a policy which outlines what steps you can take when discriminatory behaviour persists after you have told them that it is unacceptable. The next step usually involves giving a written warning setting out types of behaviour that will no longer be tolerated. You do have a right to withdraw care but only with the backing of senior hospital managers.

CO-WORKERS

Do also bear in mind that most racism experienced by nurses comes from co-workers rather than patients or senior managers (Das Gupta 2009). It is quite clear within the Nursing and Midwifery Council (NMC) code that 'You must treat your colleagues fairly and without discrimination' (NMC 2008). Unfortunately, filling the gaps in the health service with internationally sourced nurses has revealed some alarming discriminatory practices within the UK. These include questioning of competence, giving special negative attention if mistakes are made and stereotyping (Allen and Larson 2003). This is more likely to be because the nurse is a foreigner or has a different cultural background than because of their colour or ethnicity.

Take action to ensure this does not happen within your team. Staff may resent the concept of recruiting from overseas. It does not help if they are seen as receiving better treatment than UK nurses, but that is no reason to treat the individual nurses any differently. Your role as a manager is to give overseas nurses the same treatment as any other new recruit. However, you should bear in mind that having come from another country, it will take them longer to settle in and adapt to UK working practices.

1. *Prepare your team for their arrival.* Get your staff to think how they would feel starting a new job in a different country. It usually takes at least 3 months to settle in. Allow them to make mistakes without judging them negatively. Make sure your team help them to learn from their experiences, including their mistakes.
2. *Ensure all new recruits have a minimum 2-week induction programme* (even if your organisation has already provided a programme specifically for the whole group of overseas nurses).
3. *Ensure each new nurse has at least one mentor* and that those mentors have attended awareness sessions on equality and diversity. Some organisations set up specific sessions for staff to learn about the culture of the country they have just recruited from.
4. *Make sure their personal development plan focuses on skills that they can transfer back home*, while ensuring they have the same career opportunities as the rest of your staff.
5. *Don't ever indulge in discussions* about 'the overseas nurses' where *they* are stereotyped by remarks such as 'good workers, never complain, a bit slow, not very assertive, etc.'. Remember, no two individuals are the same, no matter what country they come from.

UNSAFE STAFFING LEVELS

PRIORITISE PATIENT SAFETY

Nurses, unlike many other professions, work to *minimum* safe staffing levels rather than *maximum* levels. Very few wards or departments are in a position where they can ever exceed their minimum staffing levels. This means that when someone goes off sick, you need bank or agency staff to cover. But there may be situations when:

● more than one member of staff phones in sick
● there are not enough bank or agency staff to cover
● members of staff call in sick or are sent home during the course of a shift
● the workload suddenly and unexpectedly increases beyond your team's capacity to provide the required patient care.

Most will be familiar with the following actions to take in such circumstances:

1. Inform a senior manager to see if staff can be moved from elsewhere in the hospital.
2. Phone around for staff to come in. Most wards and departments keep a list of staff home numbers which will be used in such emergencies. (Remember that this is confidential information and must be kept locked away.)

3. Inform all relevant managers of the situation, including the bed manager, to ensure that patients are admitted elsewhere, and cancel any further admissions where possible.
4. Fill in an incident form.

Once every avenue has been attempted, some nurses forget the most important last step; to *prioritise*. If your workload is far greater than your capacity to deliver, do not tell your staff to just do what they can. That is tantamount to muddling through and is dangerous. Important things may be missed.

Ensure your team take some time after handover to work out with their team what care is essential and what is desirable (i.e. can be left) for that shift. When very short staffed, maintaining the patients' safety becomes a greater priority than the provision of a high standard of care. Your team should be able to decide among themselves issues such as:

● which patients need a full blanket bath and which patients can just make do with a hands and face wash
● which patients' wound dressings can be left until the next shift
● any administration that does not affect individual care such as audits and unnecessary form filling *will* be left undone.

These must be conscious decisions and not left to chance. Don't expect your staff to do everything as if normally staffed saying that it is fine if things get missed or mistakes get made. Short staffing is not an excuse for mistakes.

Keep the patients and relatives informed, put up a notice saying something like, 'We have three staff on today instead of the required five due to high sickness levels. Please bear with us. We have had to prioritise in order to maintain essential levels of care. If you wish to speak to a nurse, it would be helpful for us if it could wait until this afternoon or tomorrow unless your request is urgent'. A notice such as this will make sure that your patients and their relatives are still confident in your management skills despite the fact that you are obviously short staffed.

PUT EVERYTHING IN WRITING

Inform your line manager not only about the situation but also what you and your team have decided in terms of the care that is to be administered and which aspects of care will be left undone in order to maintain basic safe standards for all patients. Confirm the situation and the decisions that you made via an e-mail to the appropriate manager. If the situation happens when you are not on duty, make sure your team know to take such actions, keep written notes and inform the appropriate people of their decisions.

Try not to fill in the shift yourself each time unless absolutely necessary, and don't expect your staff to either. Part of your role as a manager is to ensure that your team are fit and well, and maintain a good work/life balance, not to work them to exhaustion. Your role is to look ahead and deal with the cause of the short staffing, not to continually 'plug the gaps'.

INCIDENT FORMS

You are usually required to fill in an incident form each time your team are subject to dangerously low staffing conditions. It is good to ensure that the situation is being noted but incident reporting is not taking action; it is simply monitoring the situation. Do not just write who has been informed in the section entitled 'Action taken'. Write what action you have taken in terms of the priorities you have made with your team and your decisions about what will not be done. If the number of slips, trips and falls increases due to shorter levels of staffing, you will be able to prove via the incident forms that you have done everything in your power to prevent this.

CLIQUES

Despite your best intentions, you may find that cliques form within your team, particularly if you have members of staff who have been with you for many years. These long-term employees can be invaluable in terms of stability and maintaining high standards. They tend to be loyal and can become almost like part of a family. However, it can have a detrimental effect, especially with newcomers to the team who find it difficult to fit in.

EFFECTS ON NEW RECRUITS

Cliques can result in the loss of self-confidence of a new member of staff. Their work may suffer and you could find you have a new staff nurse who is not quite living up to your initial expectations. Worse still, they may leave within a few months for another job but not tell you the real reason; in fact, they may not realise the reason themselves. If someone does not fit in to a new work environment, they tend to blame themselves for not having the right social skills. Few may admit that to their manager, so you will be left in the dark as to the real reason. Try and be alert to the signs.

BREAKING UP A CLIQUE IN YOUR TEAM

Cliques that are causing problems within your team need to be broken up. There are several ways you can do this. The first and most obvious is to arrange the roster so that they do not always work together. When they are on duty together, encourage them to take different breaks as much as possible. Another option is to select one or two members of the clique and give them specific tasks or projects for which they must report to you. Give them lots of encouragement, praise and rewards for a job well done. This helps to divide them from the rest of the group. A similar result may be gained if you ensure that each time you recruit a new member of staff, you assign one member of the clique to be their mentor. Give the mentor lots of positive feedback around their work with the newcomer.

PROMOTION TO WARD MANAGER WITH THE SAME TEAM

You may find that when you become a ward manager it could well be on the same ward where you have been in a senior staff nurse or deputy ward manager role. You will be in the unenviable position of managing staff whom you have been working alongside very well for some time. You may find that they are happy with the situation and continue to work well as a team. However, be mindful of new members coming into the team; you could unwittingly become part of a clique. This happens so easily.

So, if your first ward manager's post is on the same ward with the same team, it is advisable to take the following actions:

1. *Create a space between you and your previous colleagues.* This can be achieved by making sure that you give equal time to every single member of the team, including time spent with each one on lunch breaks.
2. *Never talk about personnel issues with the long-term staff,* even if you have known and worked alongside them for years. You are now their manager and it is not professional to do so. If you do, they will feel privileged compared to the others and the rest of the team will feel left out. It creates divisions within the team which you should avoid at all costs. Making sure you are not part of any clique is very important. You need to set the tone for how you expect your team to behave and model it.

WHAT IF YOUR OWN LINE MANAGER IS PART OF A CLIQUE?

You may find yourself in a situation where you are managing a team that has worked together for years and which includes your own line manager. They may even have trained together. This is not an uncommon situation, but you must take control of it. Do not let your position be undermined by letting your staff bypass you and going to your line manager, who also happens to be an old friend of theirs, about issues pertaining to your ward.

If your line manager is taking time to listen to your staff concerns and starting to intervene without involving you, tell them how damaging the situation is. They may think that they are helping you out by listening to their friends/old colleagues and reporting back to you, but this can be more of a hindrance than a help. Agree on a joint strategy with your line manager about what action you would prefer to be taken when a member of your team goes to them; i.e. refer that person back to you and do not take the time to listen to the concerns until that staff member has spoken with you first.

If your line manager allows the clique to continue and you find them liaising with your team and not involving you, you could try explaining the situation to their line manager and asking for their intervention. Whatever you do, don't let the situation continue. It can gradually erode your confidence in your ward management skills and could be quite damaging for team morale.

BE SPECIFIC ABOUT EXPANDING NURSING ROLES

'Nursing is, apparently, what nurses do and nurses do whatever on earth needs doing ... We don't always have to change nursing to fit the world's needs. Sometimes it's the things going on around it that need to change' (Radcliffe 2005). In other words, stop allowing nurses to continually take on extra roles just because someone else says it is needed. Extra roles should be taken on because it improves the patient care process and *causes no extra burden* for the staff. 'Expanding roles' is an area where as a manager you need to be proactive. It is not advisable to allow some staff to take on extra roles and other staff not to, because this can cause great divisions within your team. One example is intravenous cannulation and venepuncture. If you allow your nurses individually to decide whether or not to undertake training, you may find that:

- those nurses who can cannulate and 'take blood' have to undertake it for all the patients and not just their own
- doctors will resent the nurses who do not cannulate or 'take blood' and will be less willing to undertake what they come to see as the nurses' role
- the nurses who do not cannulate or 'take blood' will resent those who do, because they feel they are doing doctors' work and not their own
- patients will see nurses that do not cannulate or 'take blood' as less experienced.

Before you allow any extra role to be taken on in your area, discuss it as a team first. Go through the advantages and disadvantages of the added responsibility. Decide together as a team whether to embrace the new role or reject it. It you decide to embrace it, then all members of the team must train and use the skills in practice.

DEVELOP GUIDELINES

Develop guidelines with the staff so that all agree the boundaries. For example, you may only wish to cannulate patients out of hours, because that is when the service is really needed and perhaps causes less disruption to the nurses' workload. The key to deciding whether to take on the role is to ask yourselves: 'Is the main reason for taking on this extra task to maximise the nurses' role or to minimise someone else's role?'

Guidelines are less prescriptive than policies. Guidelines provide parameters within which your staff may practise safely. You should also clearly identify what the training needs are. Make sure you have the support of your organisation when taking on any expanded role in terms of hospital-wide policies or guidelines on the subject. If you develop your own local ones, make sure they are validated by the standards committee so that you are protected through your organisation's vicarious liability. The law as it currently stands provides no barriers to the expanded role; it just requires nurses to be competent. The nurse only breaches their duty of care if the care falls short of what expert professionals would define as 'reasonable'.

As always, when you decide together with your team of staff to take on an extra role, you should also agree who will cover the work that you will not be able to do in order to take on the extra role.

BE PROACTIVE WITH ENFORCED MOVES OR MERGERS OF SERVICES

It is widely recognised that in order to successfully reorganise, all staff should be given the opportunity to contribute and be involved in the changes. In other words, if your ward or department needs to be moved, merged or restructured in any way, your managers should ensure that you and your staff are fully consulted and involved in making that decision, including the consideration of all alternatives.

GET INVOLVED

Unfortunately you may find that you were not involved in making the decision. Some senior managers focus more on the outcome than the process, of which communication and staff involvement are a great part. However, don't always blame the hospital board of directors or your managers if decisions are made without your involvement. You should also bear some of the blame. If you were making full use of your networking and political awareness skills, you would probably have ensured your involvement to some extent. If you decide to concentrate on running your own department without involving yourself in what else is going on within the organisation, you will be left out. So if you find yourself in such a situation, look at the skills and networks you need to develop to ensure it never happens again (see Ch. 9).

PLAN AHEAD

In the meantime, if you do suddenly find that your service is going to be restructured, you must plan ahead for this change. Even a relatively small change like moving your team to a different ward or site or merging with another team can result in long-lasting problems if not handled correctly. Staff morale can plummet, people will look elsewhere for jobs and the standard of care may well fall.

First, find out why the restructuring is required and explain the facts to your team. Take care not to procrastinate, backbite or talk negatively about the decision in front of your team. If you disagree with the enforced change, make your feelings known to your managers but only if you can offer a realistic alternative solution. If you cannot, you will have to accept the decision and then focus on your main objectives, which are:

● supporting, involving and developing your team
● maintaining a good standard of patient care.

Develop a project plan with your team to manage the move or merger. Don't accept a plan developed by more senior managers. Only you and your staff will be able to identify and plan the finer details. Present the final project plan to your manager or, better still, involve your manager in the development of the plan.

DEVELOPING A PROJECT PLAN

So how do you develop a project plan? This is far easier than it sounds. The following steps will help you in the process:

1. Find out what your deadline is for completing the move or merger.
2. Inform your team as soon as possible. Take time to listen to their concerns and explain why the decision has been made. Make sure all valid concerns are relayed back to your manager in writing.
3. Visit the area you are moving to or meet the manager of the team you will be merging with.
4. Hold a team meeting for your staff in which you:
   — brainstorm with all your team what issues need to be considered (e.g. equipment, extra skills that staff may need) and define the tasks that need to be undertaken
   — break up the tasks into different phases, usually in terms of weeks (e.g. week 1, week 2, week 3, etc.)
   — compile a simple Gantt chart (see Appendix 13.1)
   — for each task, determine what needs to be done and by whom.

If you are merging with another team, hold the above meeting with both teams together.

5. Set dates for regular review meetings with the team to review progress against the Gantt chart and identify any problems or issues that need further attention.

Always remember that you can never communicate enough in such situations. With a team covering 24 hours per day, 7 days per week, you cannot communicate through team meetings alone. Use every other method open to you such as the ward communication book, handovers, staff notice board, etc.

INVOLVE THE EXPERTS FROM THE BEGINNING

Involve your finance manager in all stages of the plan to ensure that staff time and resources are appropriately costed and accounted for. Extra funding is usually allocated to assist with any move or merger – make sure that it is appropriately utilised.

Involve your HR manager early if staff roles are changing. They will advise on the appropriate consultation and involvement of union representatives. Don't leave all this to your manager. You are the best person to lead the process. You understand the needs of your staff and patients better than anyone else. Your manager's role is to help, support and guide you through the process.

ACTION POINTS

- If you have difficulties with your manager, start thinking about the situation from their perspective and take positive steps to improve your working relationship.
- Read through your organisation's bullying and harassment policy and familiarise yourself with what is classed as 'unacceptable behaviour'.
- Take all staff complaints seriously to avoid the need for formal grievances to be made. If a formal grievance is made, read the policy and take action quickly to remain within the tight timescales of the policy.
- Concentrate on developing the skills of your staff to deal with problematic senior health care professionals.
- Be aware and deal appropriately with any forms of discrimination, particularly towards your staff from patients, relatives or other members of your team.
- Ensure your team are aware of their responsibilities regarding equality and diversity.
- Make sure your staff formally prioritise and make sure their decisions are relayed to the appropriate line manager in writing when staffing levels are unsafe.
- Break up cliques using the roster and allocating members of the clique to orientate new recruits. Devise a joint strategy with your own line manager to break up a clique if your line manager is involved.
- Decide jointly with your staff which expanded nursing roles you will all undertake, ensuring the appropriate training and guidelines are available.
- Develop a project plan and Gantt chart with your team to help deal with any major changes, such as a ward move or merger.
- Do not ignore problematic colleagues. Take appropriate action now.

References

Allen, H., Larson, J.A., 2003. 'We need respect': experiences of internationally recruited nurses in the UK. Report presented to the RCN, University of Surrey. Online. Available: http://www.rcn.org.uk/_data/assets/pdf_file/0008/78587/002061.pdf Feb 2012.

Das Gupta, T., 2009. Real nurses and others: racism in nursing. Fernwood Press, Halifax.

Nursing and Midwifery Council, 2008. The NMC code of professional conduct: standards for conduct, performance and ethics for nurses and midwives. NMC, London.

Radcliffe, M., 2005. Rear view. Nurs. Times 101 (223), 120.

APPENDIX 13.1

EXAMPLE OF SIMPLE GANTT CHART FOR WARD MOVE/ MERGER

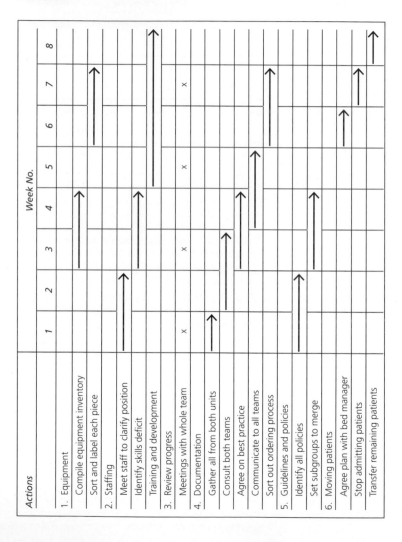

MANAGE DIFFICULT TEAM MEMBERS

If you are having problems dealing with inappropriate behaviour from members of your team, you need to look first at your style of leadership. Have you established team objectives? Are you really listening to your team and providing them with regular feedback on their performance? Do you know them well and do you spend time enhancing their individual strengths within the team? If not, go back to Chapter 3 and review your own leadership style before you focus on dealing with the individual problems.

However, despite your excellent leadership skills, there may be the occasional instance when individuals in your team do behave in an unacceptable manner.

These situations need to be dealt with swiftly. Be clear of your standards. Don't avoid the situation and don't let the individual(s) avoid you. The rest of the team will be watching you to see what you do. They will not respect a leader who ignores episodes of inappropriate behaviour.

STAFF WHO REFUSE TO LOOK PROFESSIONAL OR WEAR PROPER UNIFORM

If members of your team are deliberately flouting the uniform policy or dress code, it can be a sign of rebelliousness. Think first and foremost; is there any reason why they may wish to rebel against you? Disobedient behaviour is usually triggered when an individual feels that:

- they are not listened to
- their work is not fulfilling
- they have a controlling manager.

If you have shared objectives, listen and give regular feedback and know your staff well, there should be little reason for individuals to want to rebel (see Ch. 3). But if you are having problems despite these measures, it is advisable to take action before the rest of the team follow suit and also start flouting the uniform policy. Staff members who refuse to dress appropriately for the job may be feeling unable to express themselves in any other way.

So what do you do? First, don't just tell them what the dress code is; you can be fairly certain they will know what the policy entails. The best way to approach them is to ask about their behaviour. There will always be an underlying reason. Getting that reason to the surface depends on your questioning and listening abilities:

- 'Why are you wearing trainers/jewellery?'
- 'Why have you stopped tying your hair up?'

You may find you open a can of worms with answers such as:

- 'I don't feel we should be dictated to as to what we wear.'
- 'We are not at school any more, and I object to being treated like a child.'

These sorts of answers should be explored with further questioning. A simple 'why do you feel like that?' would suffice. They may wish to make a statement, so allow them to make it. Empathise with their predicament and support them to take action in another way.

Explain the rationale behind the policy, and the effects that their behaviour may be having on patients and others, such as decreasing people's confidence in their skills, patients' health and safety being compromised or exposing vulnerable people to an increased risk of infection.

IS IT AN INDIVIDUAL ISSUE?

If there is only one individual involved, make sure the discussion is held in private. People who want to make a statement may feel they have won if they feel that others have taken notice, or that they have got something in return for behaving this way. Once you have listened to their issue, agree appropriate alternative action and ensure they agree to abide by the terms of the policy in future. Make sure they are aware that if they continually breach the uniform policy or dress code, they are liable to disciplinary action. Remember to let them know that you will be making a file note of the discussion and agreed actions (see Ch. 4).

IS IT A TEAM ISSUE?

If you have recently taken over a new team as a ward manager, you may find yourself confronted with several members or even the whole team who are not adhering to the uniform policy. It can be a tricky situation if they have been doing this for years. It would be advisable in such a situation to raise the issue at a team meeting and have a general discussion about dress codes and uniform issues.

CULTURAL, RACE AND RELIGIOUS REQUIREMENTS

While all staff should adhere to the uniform policy, you must be sensitive to the needs of different cultures, races and religions. You should be able to accommodate these needs within the uniform policy. If there are particular difficulties, consult your human resources (HR) advisor. It would not be appropriate to discipline staff for non-compliance from having to adhere to a particular cultural, race or religious dress code.

STAFF WHO REFUSE TO ACCEPT CHANGE

Some staff members are so set in their ways that they can be rather obstinate when you want to change something at work. Remember that most people don't like change and that we all (generally) would like to keep the status quo. In the majority of cases, people who refuse to change are doing so because they have not been consulted or involved in identifying the need for the change. Keeping your team fully *informed* at each stage is not sufficient, they must be fully *involved* at each stage of the process.

If, for example, you wish to implement bedside handover where previously you have been using the office only, you cannot expect your staff to simply conform even if you have explained your rationale and the advantages many times over. The key to implementing something like this effectively is to start right at the beginning by analysing the original problem with your team. In other words, get them together and look at what is wrong with the current system before you start suggesting the solution. Bedside handover is a solution. Do the team have a problem with the office handover? If so, what do they suggest should be done? Everyone will have different views; they must be listened to. If you do come to an agreement to think about a change such as bedside handover, it's a good idea to explore the concept first with your team. SWOT analysis is a common tool used in health care for analysing the need for change within a team.

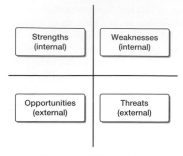

Fig. 14.1 SWOT analysis.

SWOT ANALYSIS

SWOT stands for 'strengths, weaknesses, opportunities and threats'.
Draw a matrix (Fig. 14.1) and get your team to identify:

- the strengths and weaknesses of your current system (internal)
- the opportunities and threats which may affect any future system (external).

Appendix 14.1 gives an example of a SWOT analysis. This tool helps teams to identify the weaknesses and threats of either the current system or the new system being proposed. But don't leave it there, otherwise you will just be left with a long list of factors and no attempt to do anything about it.

Getting your team to 'own' the solution

Your next step is to identify with the team what can be done to overcome the weaknesses and threats and make the most of your strengths and forthcoming opportunities. Only when you have all reached agreement about what needs to be done should you begin the process of planning and implementing the change. Doing it this way round will reduce the chances of staff refusing to change. If anyone does not want to change, they should be encouraged to come up with a valid alternative solution. You should have given them ample opportunity to do this at your initial meeting.

Remember to make sure that all members of your team have the opportunity to take part. Keep notes of the meeting and make sure everyone gets to see them.

STAFF WHO CAN'T SEEM TO PRIORITISE THEIR WORK

Some staff will continually stay late in order to:

- complete their evaluations
- finish off a task that could easily be delegated to someone else
- see to other patients whom they have neglected by concentrating on giving a high standard of care to a select few patients.

People like this tend to be perfectionists. They may lose track of time and priorities by continually striving to maintain high standards of care. However, in this day and age with higher patient turnover, increasingly complex care requirements and continual staff shortages, maintaining exceptionally high standards of care all the time is not always realistic.

Sometimes people have to be given permission to lower their standards in order to ensure that patients receive adequate care rather than receiving the ideal standard of exceptional care. If you allow them to continue striving to achieve these exceptionally high standards, it will result in either:

1. They become exhausted and end up going off sick or leaving, or
2. Some patients receive exceptionally high standards of care at the expense of others.

GETTING STAFF TO MANAGE THEIR TIME MORE EFFECTIVELY

Don't be tempted to send people on time management courses unless the course is particularly aimed at clinical staff. Time management courses are usually more helpful for office workers or people who do not spend their working days dealing with the unpredictable. Teaching people to manage their time at work becomes a lot more complex where unpredictable patient care is involved.

A more effective method of helping this individual would be to take some time to work alongside them, preferably for whole shifts at a time. That way you (or one of the more senior members of your team) can show them how to prioritise their work and how to deal with the unpredictable. Your seniority will also give them permission to lower their standards when necessary, such as in times of staff shortages. An example is helping a patient with partial paralysis from a recent stroke to get dressed. A high standard of care would be:

- to encourage the patient to do things for themselves throughout the process
- to spend time talking through the techniques they use, giving positive feedback and corrections where necessary
- to discuss any worries or concerns they may have
- to only physically intervene when absolutely necessary.

However, rehabilitation takes a lot of time and patience. If the nurse has eight patients in a similar position, delivering an exceptionally high standard of care for every one of them may simply not be feasible within the time limits of their shift. They can either give all eight an adequate standard of care, i.e. talk the patient through some of the process and physically help them through the rest, or purposefully delay some parts of their care until the later shift comes on duty.

PREVENT BURNOUT

Many nurses have learned how to manage their time and priorities through experience, but some are reluctant to lower their standards and end up exhausted by not taking their breaks or staying on late to finish their work. People who work like this rarely complain. They simply get on with it, thinking that they have to make sacrifices in order to deliver a high standard of care. Watch for people like this and take action before you end up with an exhausted and stressed member of staff. Often it is their home life and self-esteem that suffers long before the stress and exhaustion become an issue at work. By the time they reach the stage of taking time off sick from 'burnout', it may be too late for you to take action.

By spending time working with the individual as outlined above, you can show them how to work out which aspects of their work are the real priorities and which are their own personal priorities. You cannot just tell people how to plan and prioritise their care at the beginning of the shift; things always change. A patient's condition may unexpectedly deteriorate or there may be unexpected admissions or transfers. If you work the whole shift with them, you can demonstrate how to re-prioritise as changes occur.

MAINTAINING GOOD STANDARDS OF CARE

While it is advisable to ensure staff do not exhaust themselves maintaining unrealistically high standards, don't become too complacent about lowering standards of care to fit in with increasing demand. It should not come to be seen as normal practice. If your workload is increasing, make sure you are doing something about getting more staff added to your establishment to deal with the extra work, or working differently (e.g. reducing the paperwork). If staffing shortages are becoming a regular occurrence, you should be working closely with your manager to either find ways of changing or reducing the workload or increasing your staffing levels. You cannot sustain high workload with low staffing levels for any length of time without reducing standards and safety.

STAFF LABELLED AS LAZY

People may slip into what appear to be 'lazy' habits when they see their work as boring or unrewarding. They may slow down at work, perpetuate gossip and spend time on less important tasks rather than the ones that really matter.

People who are labelled as 'lazy' appear to be getting away with doing as little work as possible. This is usually because of one of three things:

1. Lethargy due to physical or mental illness.
2. Heavy personal life/non-work commitments.
3. Lack of motivation.

Before you take action, try and identify which one of the three it is. If the laziness is intermittent, then it may be because they lack motivation. If it is a permanent feature, there may be an underlying cause, such as illness. If it is because of poor physical or mental health (e.g. stress, depression or a long-term back problem), consider a GP referral, or a referral to the occupational health department for advice. Some time off sick may be all that is needed to recuperate.

If there are difficulties juggling family commitments with work, find out what you can do to facilitate adapting working hours around family life, such as:

● more flexible shift patterns
● different start and finish times
● temporary reduction in working hours.

You may feel that the family life of staff members is their own problem but such an attitude is unwise. Your role as a manager is to enable your team to provide their best efforts. Give less to your team and your team will give less to you. Whatever you do, you cannot ignore this issue with individual members of staff, especially when they continue to be paid the same as their colleagues for providing less work. It could lead to resentment from the rest of your team.

On the other hand, if a staff member thinks nothing of going out 'clubbing' between late and early shifts, they obviously do not value or appreciate their responsibilities as part of your team. This may well be a sign that they lack motivation at work.

DEALING WITH THOSE WHO LACK MOTIVATION

People who are lazy for reasons other than illness or overwhelming personal responsibilities have discovered a way of not doing something that they don't want to do. Spending time talking to someone or persistently 'telling them off' because of their perceived laziness generally doesn't help. Their experience shows them that doing more is not in their best interests, so why should they change? The rewards for doing less work are probably far more preferable to the consequences of being reprimanded. Lazy people are clever people; you should try and channel this cleverness into areas that do interest them.

Find out how you can motivate them: it's all part of being a good leader – knowing what makes each individual in your team tick and taking time to work on those motivators (see p. 50). The unfortunate thing about managing people in health care is that you cannot provide monetary rewards, but there are other ways. Giving good feedback in front of others helps. Find out what part of their role they like and ensure they get to do this part only if they complete the 'boring' part. Reward-based systems have their place.

This is all about work/life balance. Whether the person is working too hard or playing too hard, the critical thing for you as their manager is to get them to re-evaluate and redress the imbalance.

ARE THEY IN THE RIGHT JOB?

If a member of your staff cannot summon up any enthusiasm at all for their job then it might be best to encourage them to consider whether this is the right job for them. If the work in your ward is not stimulating for them, despite your best efforts, then perhaps they are working in the wrong environment. Don't take this personally. Work with them to find out where their skills lie and what they really want to do, then help them towards that goal. Help to provide them with the appropriate training and development for their chosen role, and provide assistance with job applications, interviews and references on condition that they pull their weight at work in the meantime. At the very least, you are providing them with the required motivation to stop being lazy while they remain with you looking for another job.

STAFF WITH ALCOHOL PROBLEMS

STAFF WHO TURN UP FOR DUTY DRUNK

What do you do when a member of staff turns up for duty who is obviously under the influence of alcohol? The answer is simple: send them home again. This can only be done by someone who is the person's direct line manager. If you are not on duty, the nurse-in-charge should consult with your line manager or whoever is on call. That manager will then make the decision to send the staff member home. There is usually no need to suspend the member of staff from duty or prevent their return the next day or when their next shift is due. Suspension of staff is only required if there is a risk of potential harm to patients or staff (or themselves).

The next step is up to you. For example, if this was a one-off incident and the member of staff is a competent worker with a previously unblemished record, you may decide to end the matter with a 'telling off' on their return. This goes against most policies but may help to maintain the morale and respect of both the individual and the rest of the team. Remember, a good leader will take risks and endeavour to cut through red tape and bureaucracy.

If you decide to follow the formal policy route, you should instigate a formal investigation into the incident. This is often done by an HR advisor, but could be anyone who is unrelated to the incident. They will interview all witnesses and formal statements will be taken. The staff member who was sent home will also be interviewed as part of the investigatory process. This gives them a chance to give their side of the story. Remember to ensure that any members of staff who are interviewed and required to give formal statements are informed of their rights to have a trade union representative, colleague or friend present. Some investigators forget this very important part of the process.

The person appointed to carry out the investigation will gather all the evidence together in the form of a report and make recommendations. It all needs to be done as soon as possible after the event. The recommended action will depend on whether it is the individual's first offence (usually a verbal or written warning) or whether their actions were serious and detrimental to patient care (written warning or dismissal).

If it is not the first offence or the offence is of a more serious nature

If this is not the first time that this has happened or the person's actions were serious and detrimental to patient care, then you should not hesitate to follow the policy route. The investigation report may recommend a disciplinary hearing. It may also recommend that you provide further support or help for the person's drinking/personal problems. Your manager will make that decision and will lead the disciplinary panel where they will have the option to issue a formal verbal or written warning. If the circumstances surrounding the incident were very serious and compromised patient care, your manager could make a decision to dismiss at the disciplinary hearing.

STAFF WHO HAVE A LONG-TERM DRINK PROBLEM

Managing substandard work or misconduct due to prolonged alcoholism is an entirely different process. You usually have the option of using any one of the three following procedures, depending on the circumstances:

1. Disciplinary procedure.
2. Capability or competency procedure.
3. Sickness/absence procedure.

There may also be a drugs/alcohol policy that you would need to refer to. Always consult your HR advisor, who will guide you as to which policy is most appropriate.

You should offer reasonable support if any members of staff admit that they have a problem with alchohol or drugs and who are prepared to make a concerted effort to overcome this. Your role is to treat these staff with sympathy and in complete confidence. Make sure you involve the occupational health department at an early stage. Part of your support process should include the granting of leave to see their GP or attend counselling sessions. Such action will be considered in the event of disciplinary action but will not be seen as an alternative to disciplinary action if it is deemed necessary.

In any event, be aware that your prime concern is the protection of the patients. If any registered nurse fails in their duty of care towards their patients due to the influence of alcohol, you can dismiss them at a disciplinary hearing and you may also be obliged to recommend their removal from the register.

MEMBERS OF STAFF WHO DON'T GET ON

Allowing personal differences to get in the way of work is unprofessional and should not be tolerated. Since you are the one who is responsible for creating the right environment for good teamwork, you have a big role to play when members of your team don't get on. If left unattended to, the situation can end up affecting the whole team. You must step in at once or other members of the team will begin choosing sides. Those not caught up in the conflict will look to you to resolve it. They will see it as a failure on your part if you allow the situation to continue.

Five suggested steps to resolving conflict within your team immediately are the following:

1. Bring the two team members into your office to work together on some sort of solution. Give them each some time to explain their position. They need to know that you have given them the chance to air their grievances. Don't

give them more than 5–10 minutes each. You are there as a manager, not a counsellor. Don't let them interrupt each other, find fault or try to apportion blame.

2. Once they have explained their sides, ask each in turn to say what they feel the other person should do differently. Make sure their solutions are clear and 'do-able'. Something like 'I want her to change her attitude' is too general and doesn't get you anywhere. Get them to be more specific; get them to say exactly what they want the other person to stop doing, such as 'I want her to stop pulling a face and walking off whenever I ask her to help me with something'. Then get each in turn to say what they want the other person to do instead, such as 'I want her to tell me straight if she is unhappy with what I have asked her to do and why'.

3. When these actions have been clarified, get each side to commit to doing at least one of the suggested solutions. Get them to agree to give each other feedback and acknowledge times when the other person has made the effort to change. This gets both parties to focus on the positive side of things.

4. Let them know in no uncertain terms that it is down to them to make this work. If they do not make the effort and allow the situation to continue, inform them that you will have no choice but to take formal action.

5. Make a brief file note of the discussion, including an outline of the agreed actions. Let them read it through and sign if necessary. Give each of them a copy.

Following this discussion, make it a priority to observe them closely over the next few weeks. Give positive feedback when you notice a change in their behaviour. Hopefully the situation will resolve. However, if it does not improve within a few weeks (don't leave it any longer), bring them both into your office again and outline the formal route that you will take should you see no improvement over the next couple of weeks. Again, make another file note.

Hopefully, the situation will be resolved following the second meeting. But if it is not, you will have no choice but to take the formal route. This is usually the disciplinary policy but check first with your HR advisor, who will point you in the direction of any other appropriate policy that you may have within your organisation.

STAFF WHO SEEM CARELESS AND SLOPPY

It can be really frustrating when dealing with members of staff who don't give enough attention to the important details when caring for patients. Their work may be hurried and sloppy but they may seem quite content and think that they are doing fine. Some people tend to make lots of mistakes but don't seem to see it as a problem. Important observations may not be done, discharge arrangements will be left for the next shift or patients requiring rehabilitation will be washed and dressed with no attention paid to assisting them to help themselves. They seem to find paying attention to detail as tiresome and dull.

One of the problems with having someone like this in your team is that it can cause resentment among the rest of the staff who constantly have to pick up the pieces. If you don't do anything about it, you are effectively sanctioning their behaviour. They could be perfectly happy to continue, while thinking that the rest of the team are at fault for making such a fuss.

USE OF COMPETENCY PACKAGES

Usually these types of people need to be told to slow down and take more responsibility for their patient care. You have to reiterate what the expected standards are. However, just saying this may not be sufficient. If the member of staff is junior and inexperienced, it may be a simple case of allocating a mentor to work through a competency package with them.

If the individual in question is more senior and experienced, why not get them to *develop* competences or *review* the competency package that you already have in place. Make sure that the areas of care being overlooked are included in the package. For example, if your area cares for patients requiring rehabilitation, do the competences specify how to assist the patients to help themselves rather than do everything for them? Does it assess the person's knowledge of when and why observations should be carried out? Does it set out each stage of the discharge process that should be covered and when?

Helping to write these standards down in the form of competences usually helps to stimulate the member of staff about the quality of care they are expected to provide rather than what they have got away with over the years. You may prefer to do this as part of a team meeting or discussion to help raise standards generally across the team.

USE OF POSITIVE FEEDBACK TO ENHANCE GOOD BEHAVIOUR

Reward the individual for when they have paid attention to detail by giving frequent positive feedback. When the work has not been done, get them to go back and correct or finish their work where possible. They need to learn that there are consequences for not producing an adequate standard of work.

Be prepared to stick at it. Members of staff who are careless and sloppy in their work will not change overnight. They have to unlearn their habits and acquire new ones, which takes time. If, after 3–6 months, you find that they have really not changed their ways, you should question their capability for undertaking the role. Most organisations have a policy which guides you through a specific process consisting of meetings and action plans to improve a person's capability (see Ch. 4).

Ultimately, if you follow this policy, your manager could make the decision to terminate their employment if the process is unsuccessful, but you must have explored all other avenues first and kept a full record of all your actions in the form of file notes.

STAFF WHO MANIPULATE SITUATIONS FOR THEIR OWN GAIN

Some members of staff are pretty astute when it comes to getting their own way. This behaviour often becomes apparent when it has something to do with requests and the roster. There are some members of staff who do not care what effect their requests have on other staff. You may be familiar with excuses such as:

'You told me if I put the request in first then I could have it.'

'You promised me last year that I could have this weekend off.'

'I spoke to HR and they said that I could take 4 weeks' annual leave together and that you can't refuse to give it to me.'

Manipulators will often play off one person against the other. They will go to more senior people if they cannot get their own way. This is particularly rife if individuals are aware that you and your manager do not communicate well, or have any differences. Prevent this by ensuring that you never let staff know if there are problems between you and anyone else within your organisation. Manipulators are constantly on the lookout for these and will take advantage of any perceived breakdown in communications between you and your colleagues. Don't give them the opportunity.

CONFRONT THEM DIRECTLY

Often the only way to deal with these people is to confront them directly. Don't try and beat them at their own game, because that is what you will make it – a game. Tell them exactly what you think is going on; the chances are that they will be taken by surprise. Many people who do this do it as a way of life and are unaware that their behaviour might be determined as manipulation. Explain that if they had taken a more straightforward approach, and simply asked you rather than going to someone else, they could have got what they wanted without any hassle. However, as they have now gone to someone else to try and override your authority, you are seeing things in a different light and are reluctant to concede to their demands. Tell them in future they must be more direct in their approach.

Another way is to meet with the other person whom they used to try and manipulate you. Explain the situation to them and ask the manipulator to meet with you both and explain their actions, and perhaps even apologise. It could shame them into ensuring they don't do it again. Remember to acknowledge or give positive feedback in the future each time they do use a more direct approach for something they want.

DON'T BE FOOLED BY FLATTERY

Managing a ward or department can be very isolating and it is easy to be unduly influenced by a member of staff who tells you that you are wonderful, so knowledgeable, capable or the best boss they have ever worked for. Be careful of the underlying agenda. Good factual feedback should be welcomed but a quick thank you is enough and don't let it sway your judgement or treatment of that person.

LAYING THE BLAME ON YOU

With the ever-increasing emphasis on accountability within health care, you may find that some staff are reluctant to take responsibility for their mistakes. You may hear phrases such as:

'Sister said I could do this.'
'You told us that it didn't matter if we didn't do all the observations when it was busy.'
'It wasn't my fault. If you hadn't agreed to admit those extra patients, this would never have happened.'

In situations such as these, don't be tempted to go into defensive mode with replies such as:

'I did not say that.'
'When I said that I did not mean for you to go ahead and do this.'
'It's not my fault either; don't blame me.'

Don't get into a discussion about who is to blame: concentrate on what is to be done about the situation. Get people to focus on generating solutions. Then once the problem has been dealt with, discuss and agree what steps to take to ensure there is no confusion or further misunderstanding in future similar situations.

STAFF WHO MOAN AND WHINGE

There will always be people for whom nothing ever goes right. If life isn't perfect (which it never is), they feel hard done by. Life seems to be so much better for everyone else. Other people get their weekends off, get more pay, do less work, have better working conditions, etc. For some staff, anything that is less than perfect at work (and at home) is an excuse to whinge.

The thing about people who moan and whinge is that they never seem to do anything about the situation. If they did, there would be nothing to moan about. They may perceive themselves as not being able to do anything and think that the solution always lies with others referred to as 'they' and 'them'. You can easily get used to this sort of attitude and just accept that's how this person is and get on with things. The problem with having people like this on your team is that this attitude is infectious. Once someone starts moaning in the coffee room during break time, everyone will join in.

CHALLENGE PERCEPTIONS (INCLUDING YOUR OWN)

One way of dealing with such people is to review how you perceive them. Changes to systems often take place when someone is not happy with current circumstances. If nurtured, these people could become your agents for change. Whenever you catch them moaning and whinging about something, it's better not to listen and sympathise. A better response would be to ask them to suggest a solution. This may catch them by surprise, as they would probably not be used to such a response. They may be more used to getting people to agree and moan with them. People who are challenged to do something about the situation tend to stop moaning at the very least because what you are really saying is 'if you're not prepared to do anything about it, then stop moaning'.

DON'T ALLOW A PERPETUAL MOANER TO PREVENT PROGRESS

If you have an idea that you want to raise with your team, it is wise to present it to each of them individually before raising it at a team meeting. Ask for their ideas and feedback. When you eventually raise the idea at a team meeting, you can ensure that most of the team will support you. If an individual realises that they are on their own with their usual negative opinions, they will be more reluctant to relay them. If they do, then ask them and the rest of the team what an alternative solution would be. Don't dwell on any negatives; focus on the positives. Always have an answer ready for the usual negative responses (see Table 14.1).

HOLDING A NEGATIVE VIEW OF ONESELF

Some members of staff may consistently moan and whinge that they are not good enough. For example:

'Here's the work you asked me to do; it's not very good.'
'I went to that meeting for you, but I was useless. I'm no good at that sort of thing.'
'I'm too stupid/too old/not intelligent enough.'

All these sorts of comments do is demonstrate a lack of confidence. Sometimes it's done to protect them from negative feedback. If they've said it themselves then someone else is hardly likely to say it again. If you are continuously giving all members of your staff positive feedback then you will be very unlikely to hear these things. So if it is happening, question your style of leadership; are you giving enough feedback? (See p. 49).

TABLE 14.1: Sample answers for negative responses within meetings	
Negative response	*Answer*
'I don't see how it will work. They will never allow us to do that.'	'Who won't allow us to do that? Why do you think that they won't allow us to? I see no reason why not.'
'It's all been tried before and it never makes any difference.'	'Well, I'm sorry it didn't work out for you before, but this time it is different because …'
'It's always back to us. Why should we have to do all the work?'	'If you want to see things improve, then you have to make the effort. Moaning and whinging will achieve nothing, but taking action will.'

On the other hand, you may get the odd one or two people who will put themselves down in order to get people to tell them how wonderful they are. In this case, tell them if you didn't think they were good enough they wouldn't be part of your team, and you don't want to hear them talking like that again, and leave it at that.

STAFF WHO ARE CONTINUALLY LATE FOR DUTY

We've probably all done it; seethed in silence when a member of staff wanders into handover 5 or 10 minutes late. Not only that, but some even have the nerve to bring a cup of coffee in too!

THE PROBLEM WITH LATENESS

Lateness can cause huge problems within a team, but some ward managers do little, if anything, to put a stop to it. Some don't even monitor lateness. In many other areas of work, people have less need to start on time because their jobs are outcome focused. This means that as long as they get the job done, it doesn't really matter when or even where they work. But in nursing and any other jobs that involve shift work, getting to work on time has a greater importance. Arriving late results in:

- interruption and delaying of handover
- staff from the previous shift getting off late as they have to repeat everything for the latecomers
- the latecomer risking missing vital information about their patients and therefore compromising their ability to care for the patients when the previous shift goes home
- reduced morale and working relationships within the team becoming fragmented

Ignore lateness at your peril. If allowed to continue, it may become accepted as normal practice. The staff will become divided into those that are conscientious and come in on time and those that don't. Consistent lateness is a reflection of poor attitudes about work.

GETTING TO THE ROOT OF THE MATTER

If you notice that a member of staff is regularly coming to work late, you should first try to uncover the underlying causes. If they are having genuine problems getting to work on time, such as their bus timetable being incompatible with shift start times, then it is better to compromise and formally agree to a later start time. That way, working practice can change in advance to accommodate this.

If you come to the conclusion that it is simply a poor attitude to work or because some staff members are not committed, then you need to consider your leadership style again:

1. Are your team working towards shared goals?
2. Do you give feedback to each member of staff every time you work with them?
3. Do you know each individual in your team well?

If you hesitated or answered no to any of the above questions, then perhaps you need to ascertain what else you can do to provide a more motivating environment first (see Ch. 3).

FIND A SOLUTION TOGETHER

If a member of staff continues to arrive late for duty despite you having ascertained that there are no extenuating personal circumstances and you know you have done everything outlined in Chapter 3 to maintain a motivating environment, the next step is to concentrate on finding a solution *with* them. Don't continually ask them why they are late each time. If you do, you will just receive a barrage of excuses. Turn the question round to make them suggest a solution: 'Despite our previous meeting, you still turn up late for most of your shifts. What can we do about it?'

Don't allow the rest of your staff to accommodate lateness. They must not wait to give handover. Ensure they always start on time without them. Make sure they do not summarise what the latecomer has missed. They must be made to catch up themselves afterwards. They should change, but if they don't, you have two options.

Option 1: Aim towards the disciplinary process

When dealing with persistent lateness, it is essential that you keep accurate records of all episodes, including lateness from lunch breaks. You must be able to demonstrate that you have met with the staff member to determine any possible solutions and agree actions. Make sure that during your meetings you have at some stage outlined when the lateness qualifies for disciplinary action. Before you take this route, you need to show that you have fully explored all possible solutions.

Option 2: Encourage them to look at other roles where they will be stimulated

Continual lateness, despite the actions outlined above, indicates a lack of commitment to the job so perhaps it is not the right one for them. If you have a member of staff who is truly not happy in their work, they may simply be in the wrong specialty. Don't give up on them and wait for them to leave. Help them to identify what job would really stimulate them and assist them in developing the skills to be able to apply for a post in their chosen field. Whatever happens, you do not want staff leaving your ward and telling others how they hated working in your area. Helping them to attain their chosen job will see them leave on a more positive note.

PREVENTION IS BETTER THAN CURE

Make sure you have included in your induction package:

- what time shifts begin and what is considered late
- how to inform the rest of the team if they know they will be late
- when and how disciplinary action will be undertaken for lateness.

Many organisations now have some sort of code of conduct for their employees. This usually includes the above points, so inclusion of the document in the induction package may suffice. Remember also that if you expect staff to be punctual in their arrival to work then you should also meet their expectations of getting off work on time. Don't expect staff to stay late (unless you are paying them extra). Giving time back is insufficient compensation for people having to stay late (unpaid) regularly at work.

ACTION POINTS

- Ensure all members of staff adhere to the uniform policy. If any refuse, find out why and propose alternative solutions. Take the disciplinary route only when all other avenues have been exhausted.
- Involve all members of staff in all changes by presenting the initial problem first and asking for proposed solutions. Do not present the solution first.
- Do not allow any staff members to regularly stay behind to finish work or miss their breaks. Work with them if necessary to help develop prioritising skills.
- If you feel a member of your staff is 'lazy', find out first if there are any problems with illness, personal commitments or if it is simply a lack of motivation. Take action to increase their motivation either to work more efficiently or find another job.
- Be aware of the process to take should a member of staff turn up unfit for work through alcohol or drugs, so that the appropriate action is taken in any such event.
- Resolve any problems between members of your team by calling them to a meeting immediately and taking specific action. Do not allow any situation of conflict to continue.
- Use competency packages to improve the skills of junior team members. Encourage senior team members with poor standards to review the competency packages, thus improving their own skills in the process.
- Confront any staff members who try to manipulate you.
- Encourage your team to transform negative statements into positive solutions.
- Take action immediately to stop people being persistently late for duty or late back from breaks. Show the rest of your team that you will not tolerate lateness.
- Ensure your ward induction package includes a section on how staff members are expected to behave.

APPENDIX 14.1

EXAMPLE OF A SWOT ANALYSIS FOR BEDSIDE HANDOVER

Strengths (internal)	Weaknesses (internal)
Able to match names with faces	Potential problems with confidentiality
Able to scrutinise observation charts and care plans at the same time	Unable to get chance to sit down and have a cup of tea (often only chance during shift is during handover)
Able to introduce self to patient	
Patient can be fully involved	Unable to chat/catch up with colleagues
Less time hanging around waiting for office handover to finish before being able to go home	Staff don't get to know everything about every patient
	Patients may not like it

Opportunities (external)	Threats (external)
New hand-held computers being introduced for wards that use bedside handover	New flexible working policy affecting handover times
Complies with CQC standards	Forthcoming cutbacks in staffing

GET THE BEST ADVICE

Try not to rely on just one source of advice when making decisions. How do you know for sure that the person's advice is sound? How do you know they are giving you the best option? Try to seek advice from a variety of sources. That way you will be able to make a more informed decision based on as many facts and opinions as you can access. Include your team in this when you can. Enable them to have an input and influence over the decisions you have to make which affect them.

There are various departments within health care trusts to which you can go for advice. Some are under-utilised by nurse managers. As a senior person within the trust you have access to solicitors, senior professional advisors, educational advisors, counselling services, human resource advisors, computer experts and many more. You should never have to make decisions or struggle with any aspects of your work without being able to access the appropriate support.

KNOW WHERE TO GO FOR LEGAL ADVICE

SOLICITORS

NHS organisations appoint solicitors to act and advise on their behalf in respect of legal issues. If you require legal advice regarding a problem that has arisen or may arise at work, most organisations have a procedure in place through which you can access these solicitors. This procedure is there to ensure that they are not being asked the same questions from different areas within the organisation. The solicitors can usually be accessed through the person who deals with litigation and claims, known as the litigation and claims manager, legal services manager or clinical governance manager.

It is advisable to locate the appropriate person within your organisation and to keep a copy of their contact details available at all times both for you and your staff. Your director of nursing should be your first port of call for any professional issues. They have more experience and may be able to advise without calling on the solicitors.

If you have an emergency out of hours, contact the duty manager who will have access. Some solicitors provide a 24-hour helpline for advice on clinical issues, but this number would usually be restricted for the use of a 'named' senior manager or on-call managers. Some organisations hold contracts with solicitors that include free training for staff, which is well worth accessing, but often you will have to ask first. This service is not usually widely advertised.

TRADE UNION REPRESENTATIVES

Every NHS organisation has a number of trade union representatives as well as a lead steward whose role is to protect members' rights and ensure they are treated fairly. They are specifically trained for the role. They will provide help and guidance with issues concerning employment rights, discrimination, health and safety legislation and concerns about poor practices. You can also get advice regarding legal or potential legal issues directly from your local regional office.

Both the Royal College of Nursing (RCN) and UNISON provide members with online advice services where you can get information on legal issues (RCN 2011, UNISON 2011).

KNOW WHERE TO GO FOR PROFESSIONAL ADVICE

THE DIRECTOR OF NURSING

One of the key responsibilities of your nursing director is to provide professional leadership to all nurses and midwives within the organisation. They will provide advice personally or direct you to the appropriate place to find the information you require. If you have a non-clinical line manager and need advice on a professional matter, there is no reason why you cannot contact your director or deputy director of nursing directly. Use the phone if it is an emergency; otherwise use e-mail. Directors of nursing may be the most senior nurses within your organisation but they recognise that ward managers are a vital asset and will ensure you can access the appropriate professional advice and support.

Most nurse directors have at least one deputy director plus a small team of senior health care professionals to assist them in their corporate-wide role. The nursing director, together with their team, provides a support system for nurses, midwives and allied health professionals to help maintain high standards of care across the organisation.

THE NURSING AND MIDWIFERY COUNCIL

The main aim of the NMC is to ensure that registered nurses and midwives provide high standards of care, and to protect the public. This is achieved by:

- maintaining the professional register
- setting standards
- investigating and dealing with allegations of misconduct
- providing a professional advice service for nurses and midwives.

The advice service is free and confidential. It is provided by a team of professionals qualified in various specialties such as mental health nursing, paediatric nursing, adult nursing and learning disabilities. You can e-mail or call one of the professional officers with your query or access information from their Web site: http://www.nmc-uk.org.

In addition, you can access all current NMC publications such as *Raising and Escalating Concerns: Guidance for Nurses and Midwives* or *Guidance for Continuing Professional Development for Nurse and Midwife Prescribers*. These can all be downloaded free from their Web site.

UNIVERSITY LECTURERS

Your link lecturer is the obvious choice for advice regarding issues in your specialty, but there is no reason why you cannot access other university lecturers for expert advice. Most would be only too happy to provide information within their specialty. E-mail is usually the best approach to use as lecturers can be difficult to contact by phone due to their Monday to Friday working pattern and tight teaching schedules.

Keep a copy of the annual course prospectus from your local university's department of nursing studies or health and social care. This will contain all the contact details of the lecturers in each specialty. You will find most lecturers helpful in professional matters and if they do not know the answer, they will usually refer you to someone who does.

UTILISE THE CHAPLAINCY DEPARTMENT

Chaplaincy services are under-used by some ward managers. They usually offer an excellent service which involves more than just providing spiritual care to patients of various faiths. They also provide a service for staff, including those who do not profess any particular faith. The chaplaincy services can be invaluable when your team is going through a particularly hard time, such as dealing with difficult deaths or more deaths than usual. They can also be very supportive in times of staff shortages when members of your team may be distressed at being unable to meet the usual high standards of care.

BEREAVEMENT

Part of the role of the chaplaincy department is to educate staff in dealing with bereavement (Department of Health 2003). They can also provide support to members of your team who suffer a personal bereavement. However, they will not come to you; you have to access these services in times of need. It can be difficult if you do not know them very well. It is better to prepare by building up a good relationship with your chaplaincy team before you get to the stage of requesting their services.

STAFF SUPPORT

It does not matter if you or members of your staff are not religious. Hospital chaplaincy services do not impose their religious beliefs. Their role is to meet both religious and spiritual needs and they are not concerned about whether or not staff members go to church.

It would be wise to include a meeting with a member of the chaplaincy service as part of your induction programme for new members of staff (if your trust-wide induction programme does not already include this).

STAFF TRAINING AND DEVELOPMENT

Chaplains working in health care receive specialist training, education and experience in working with people in challenging situations. They can contribute to your staff training programme in a number of subjects such as:

- listening skills
- dealing with difficult situations
- appreciation of religious and cultural diversity
- advanced directives or 'living wills'.

Their skills may also be helpful in the facilitation of clinical supervision groups for your staff.

Consider inviting one of the chaplaincy team to some of your ward meetings. Their skills may be particularly useful in debriefing sessions following distressing circumstances such as serious incidents requiring investigation, accidents or mistakes.

INCREASE STAFF AWARENESS

Make sure all members of staff are fully aware of how to access the chaplaincy service and that they do not have to be religious in order to do so. Ensure they know they can call on the chaplaincy service for advice on a range of matters including advance directives (living wills), palliative care and even personal support for individual staff, including bereavement or relationship issues. The chaplains are increasingly being used as someone to talk to who will listen and help individuals to reflect in absolute confidence. They also have the advantage in that they are not part of any internal hierarchy.

Obviously it will be far easier to call on their advice if you have built up a good working relationship with them in the first place. This is what networking is all about. It is a major part of your role as a manager. It is best not to leave it until your chaplaincy service contacts you or when you feel in need of their help and assistance.

USE BUT DON'T ABUSE THE NURSE SPECIALISTS

The role of the nurse specialist varies between organisations, but overall they tend to fall into two categories:

1. Trust-wide nurse specialists.
2. Departmental nurse specialists.

The trust-wide nurse specialists usually report directly to the nursing director and have responsibility across the organisation because their area of expertise involves a large majority, if not all, of the patients. The trust-wide specialties include areas such as infection control and tissue viability. They are responsible for implementing and maintaining standards of care and monitoring performance throughout the organisation.

The departmental nurse specialists are also responsible for standards of care within their specialty across the organisation. The difference is that their specialty involves a specific group of patients. These include areas such as diabetes, respiratory and epilepsy. Their duties usually involve managing a caseload of patients, often on an outpatient basis, where they are responsible for activities such as running clinics, performing diagnostic tests and providing follow-up care and support.

DIFFERENT EDUCATION AND DEVELOPMENT RESPONSIBILITIES

The main priority for trust-wide specialists is usually the education and development of staff. Their role is to reduce common problems such as infection and pressure sores through promotion of best practice.

The main priority for departmental nurse specialists is the provision of care for their caseload of patients. They also have a responsibility for the education and development of staff within the rest of the organisation but only as and when that can be fitted around their core responsibilities. It is not their main priority, but they will do their best to be available for specialist advice and support where possible.

BE WARY OF DE-SKILLING YOUR STAFF

It has become an issue in some areas where a nurse specialist may be called as soon as a patient within their specialty is admitted. The problem here is that nurse specialists are not employed to undertake the work that a general nurse should be quite capable of doing. If, for example, a patient is admitted to a general medical ward with angina, it should not be necessary to call in a cardiac nurse specialist to provide rehabilitation advice. That should remain within the remit of the general medical nurse.

The role of the nurse specialist is to provide appropriate education and advice to enable the general nurses to improve their own skills. If members of your team fall into the habit of calling in a nurse specialist each time, they will lose their skills in that area. Your role as ward manager is to continuously improve the skills of your team. Use the nurse specialists to help you in this role by asking them to provide education and development for your team.

Develop close links with all the trust-wide nurse specialists plus those who are directly linked with your specialty. Usually the trust-wide specialist nurses will be working towards specific targets and will be only too happy to come along at your request to assist in the education and development of staff. This also helps them in achieving their targets, as do link nurse roles.

LINK NURSE ROLES

Beware of having a link nurse role for each specialist subject. Ideally each individual in your team should have no more than one link nurse role, otherwise they may not be able to make the most of the development opportunities for each subject area and they risk becoming overloaded.

There will always be more link-nurse roles than there are available nurses within your team. The key is to prioritise. Any areas linked to the quality outcome indicators should come top of the list. For example, it is advisable to have a link nurse for infection control and tissue viability. Other link nurse roles depend on the frequency of patients admitted with the specialist condition on your ward. You may find diabetes is the next key priority on a ward where a large number of patients admitted are diabetic.

If there are more link nurse roles than the number of staff in your team, get your team together and decide what your top priorities are. Make a conscious decision to leave out the rest. Inform your manager in writing (e-mail will suffice) about the decision you have made with your team and why. You may have an outcry from nurse specialists who want a link nurse on your ward to maintain communications, but the welfare of your team comes before the needs of the nurse specialist. Work together with them to find some other less time-consuming way that you can maintain communications.

HELP PATIENTS AND RELATIVES ACCESS THE RIGHT ADVICE

PATIENT ADVICE AND LIAISON SERVICE

All patients and relatives have access to advice and support in making a formal complaint about their health services, but in England, the Department of Health has gone one step further through the development of patient advice and liaison services (PALS). Every NHS organisation in England now has a PALS office employing several individuals to provide information and advice to patients and relatives about any concerns they may have while in hospital. (This service is currently unique to England: it is not available in Scotland, Wales and Northern Ireland.) The main role of PALS officers is to resolve problems and concerns quickly by liaising with health care professionals and managers on the patients' behalf. A great deal of money is spent on this service; money that could be spent on more front-line staff. Why? In part, maybe it is because health care professionals have not been listening or providing advice and information sufficient for the needs of patients and their relatives.

Having a PALS office in every NHS organisation in one sense can be seen as a poor reflection on the service we (nurses) provide, yet it is obviously needed. Some health care professionals are actually referring their patients to PALS for advice and support. Think carefully about it; if patients or relatives from your ward are having to go to PALS for information or help to resolve issues, it indicates that you and your team are not meeting their needs. If you find this is happening frequently, it is worth using one of your team meetings to review all your dealings with PALS and identify areas where you need to improve. The PALS officers keep records of all visits to enable you to learn from the information.

INFORMATION LEAFLETS

It is imperative to ensure the supply of information sheets and leaflets is always plentiful, including those on how to make a complaint. However, given the huge array of literature which is now available, try to ensure that you and your staff select the appropriate ones for individual patients' and relatives' needs rather than expect them to help themselves. Patients who are given specific leaflets (with their name written on the front) are more likely to read and take note than if they were just left to help themselves from the leaflet rack.

WARD ROUNDS

Some patients and relatives become completely 'tongue-tied' when confronted with a group of doctors standing around the bedside. It is one of the main reasons why a patient's nurse should be part of the ward round. The nurse's role is to act as the patient's advocate, encouraging them to ask questions or asking on their behalf if necessary (see p. 96).

Your staff should routinely advise patients and relatives to prepare for ward rounds and other visits by writing down their questions in advance. They should be reassured that this is normal and that the doctor (or other health care professional) would prefer this to ensure that the patients' needs have been met. Illness makes patients and relatives a lot more vulnerable than they would be normally. Don't expect them to be able to access all the right information by themselves.

KEEP UP-TO-DATE WITH RISK MANAGEMENT ISSUES

Risk management basically means taking measures to reduce the likelihood of any harm happening to your patients and staff. Managing health care delivery will always involve a degree of risk, but minimising those risks is a key part of your role.

PERFORMANCE INDICATORS FOR RISK MANAGEMENT

Your organisation will have a set of performance indicators to measure the effectiveness in the way they identify, reduce and manage risk. The main NHS performance indicators are set nationally and vary according to whether you are in England, Wales, Scotland or Northern Ireland. In England, the NHS Litigation Authority (NHSLA) has specific risk management standards against which your trust is assessed (NHSLA 2011).

It is important that you are aware of your organisation's targets for minimising risk and that your staff are trained in risk management. You should also access training for yourself in incident investigation and root cause analysis, if you have not already done so.

RISK MANAGEMENT BOARD

The chief executive has overall responsibility for meeting the statutory requirements and guidance issued by the Department of Health. Most health care organisations have a risk management board and employ a specific team of staff to ensure that you have access to the right advice and support. They also ensure the appropriate policies and procedures are in place to help you minimise clinical and non-clinical risk. Find out who is responsible for clinical governance or risk management within your organisation and make sure they become part of your network. Perhaps even shadow them for a day. Not only will you benefit from their knowledge and find out what you should be doing, but you will get to know them well enough to be able to call on them for expert advice when required. You will also get to know their team and which individuals are the best to call for advice and support.

DIRECTORATE RISK MANAGEMENT COMMITTEE

Your directorate will also have a specific group or committee which continually assesses and manages risk. This could be part of your directorate clinical governance group or you may have a separate directorate risk management group. It would be advisable to make sure you are a member of this group.

Be careful if you decide to delegate the role of risk management to a member of your team. You still remain accountable for ensuring that effective risk management measures are undertaken in your ward or department. It is advisable that you retain the role of risk management lead for your area and ensure you get regular feedback from your link staff for issues such as manual handling and health and safety. You retain overall responsibility for all risk management issues so make sure you are kept well informed to be able to ensure your systems and processes are all in order.

CONSULT POLICIES, PROCEDURES AND GUIDELINES

WHY SO MANY POLICIES?

It seems that there are policies and procedures for everything we do these days, including of course a policy for the storage and filing of policies! But looking at it positively, the more policies and procedures that your organisation has is indicative of how well employees are looked after and valued. If you have relatively few compared to other organisations, it could mean that both you and your patients are at greater risk of harm.

Policies and procedures are very important in informing your day-to-day work. They indicate what the organisation expects with regards to staff behaviour and work standards. They guide you as to what is acceptable and what is not. Without this guidance, you would have no standard with which to measure others. If members of staff produce a lower standard of work, there would be little you could do about it without the appropriate policy or procedure in place. You and your staff would also have fewer rights.

ACCESSIBILITY

Policies and procedures are useful documents and should be easily accessible on your intranet system for all staff to consult during the course of their shift. They can often be a better source of advice than seeking someone else's opinion. They not only outline good practice but they also include the most current legislation. Try to read the appropriate policy regarding any staff management issues before consulting other individuals for advice. Policies and procedures give you a good idea about the correct line of action to follow in most situations.

COMMUNICATION OF POLICY CHANGES

Whenever you receive a new, revised or updated policy, find out exactly what has been changed in the policy. You can do this by calling the person responsible for the revised policy or procedure. Once you have done this, inform all your staff. If you just tell your staff that the policy has been replaced with a new one, it is highly unlikely that anyone will have the time or inclination to read it through. However, they will take note if you highlight what the changes are either in your ward communication book or via a team meeting. Asking staff to read through whole policies and procedures is unrealistic and you know it won't happen.

EVIDENCE-BASED GUIDELINES

Ensure that evidence-based guidelines and standards are also easily accessible for your team. All clinical guidelines you use on your ward should be based on the best possible evidence. Guidelines should not just be an outline of the current practice on your ward for new members. You must make sure they are up-to-date.

However, updating guidelines takes valuable time which you and your team probably do not have. Try and use your specialist association for guidelines pertaining to your specialty and use national guidelines wherever possible. *The Royal Marsden Manual of Clinical Procedures* is an ideal example of evidence-based guidelines which are applicable for use in most areas (Dougherty and Lister 2011). Many organisations now have this available online but, if not, it is worth having a book like this available on the ward for your staff. It will save you and your staff wasting time on having to develop your own and continually having to update them.

The National Institute for Health and Clinical Excellence (NICE) guidelines are also easily accessible online (http://www.nice.org.uk/Guidance/CG/Published) and the Scottish Intercollegiate Guidelines Network (SIGN) guidelines are available in Scotland (http://www.sign.ac.uk). Both sets of guidelines are accessible for all health care professionals both in and outside the UK.

If you are really keen on developing your own, get the right help and support. Contact your organisation's practice development department. If they do not have the right expertise, they will still be able to help by finding the right person or the right information on your behalf. They will also be able to advise on how to formulate the guidelines and standards and how to get them validated.

MAXIMISE COMPUTER ACCESS

THE WORLD WIDE WEB

Nothing beats the Internet for providing instant access to information. It means that individuals do not have to leave the ward area to find the information they need to enhance their practice. There are many Web sites that you can access for up-to-date clinical information including those listed below:

1. Professional academic resources. All these are only available for NHS employees:
   — NHS Evidence (England: http://www.evidence.nhs.uk)
   — Health on the Net (Northern Ireland: http://www.honni.qub.ac.uk)
   — The Knowledge Network (Scotland: http://www.knowledge.scot.nhs.uk)
   — e-Library for Health (Wales: http://www.wales.nhs.uk/sitesplus/878).
2. RCN online library and information service: http:// www.rcn.org.uk/library. Available for RCN members only.
3. NICE: http://www.nice.org.uk/guidance.

4. SIGN: http://www.sign.ac.uk.
5. Patient information Web sites are also very useful for general information especially when you have patients admitted with conditions you are not familiar with (see p. 92).

GETTING YOUR STAFF TO USE COMPUTERS

Some nurses are still 'computer shy' and find it difficult to use computers. Try and encourage the more IT literate members of your team to help and teach those who are less so. There are also various IT courses that staff can access, including the national Essential IT Skills course in England and Northern Ireland (NHS Connecting for Health 2011). All staff (including those with good IT skills) should attend regular computer skills training not only to keep abreast of all the new IT systems being introduced, but more importantly to maintain awareness of regulations regarding the handling of confidential information, particularly with the increasing computerisation of patient records.

In addition, you should ensure there are enough computers on your ward so that one is available at all times for staff to look up information instantly without having to queue.

UTILISE THE KNOWLEDGE AND SKILLS OF YOUR NURSING COLLEAGUES

CHANNEL THE ENTHUSIASM WITHIN YOUR TEAM

As pointed out in Chapter 3, a good leader knows the strengths and weaknesses of all their team members. Work on those strengths. It you have an issue where you need more knowledge in order to make an informed decision, delegating the task of fact finding is often useful for the development of one of the individuals within your team. Don't delegate unless it serves a useful purpose for the person you are delegating to. Your junior sister/charge nurses need as much experience as they can get to prepare them for the next role. Make sure you learn together with each new experience.

MAKE FINDING INFORMATION A STAFF DEVELOPMENT OPPORTUNITY

If you come across a problem which you have never dealt with before, getting others to find out what the options are for dealing with the problem can be good experience for them as well as helping you. Don't always assume that if you don't know what to do, it's up to you to find out. You can still ask others to find out for you. Just point the individual in the right direction for finding out the information.

If, for example, you have a patient who divulges some confidential information to a member of your staff who feels that others should know about it and comes to you for advice and support, your first instinct may be to contact your trade union, your organisation's solicitors and perhaps even the NMC advice line for further information on what to do. Delegating these actions to your junior sister/ charge nurse as a learning oppportunity may be far more productive. They will feel they have accomplished something worthwhile and will be enthusiastic about the experience. If you delegate it because you do not have the time, it will quite rightly be regarded as a chore and there will be less learning from the experience.

Whenever you are confronted with staff members who have a problem, be honest: 'I have no idea what to do in this situation. Who do you think might be able to help? Try calling them to see what they advise'.

DRAW ON THE EXPERIENCE OF YOUR PEERS

Regularly meeting with other ward managers within your organisation is one way of learning from them, but it is also a good idea to set up some sort of network in between these meetings. This ensures that you have instant access to their knowledge and experience. E-mail is often the best way to do this. If you have not already done so, set up a group e-mail address of all the ward managers within your organisation and encourage them to do the same. This can prove invaluable in cases where you need urgent information. Few ward managers with the appropriate knowledge would ignore the following e-mail addressed to the group:

> 'A member of staff has come to me with an allegation of bullying from one of the agency nurses. I have not dealt with this situation before. If anyone else has experience of a similiar issue, I would be grateful to know how you handled it.'

Always remember to remain confidential and never divulge sensitive information which could result in the individuals involved being identified. You can contact each other by phone or face-to-face afterwards if details need to be discussed in depth.

USE E-MAIL

All the ward managers within your organisation would benefit by maintaining close contact and learning from each others' experiences. In the past, without e-mail, this has been difficult because of the nature of the role. Most would be reluctant to call colleagues and interrupt their work and you don't have time to keep leaving the ward to go around and talk to your colleagues. With e-mail, you do not have to leave the ward and you are not interrupting your colleagues in the course of their work. In addition, e-mail takes up far less time and is a lot more succinct.

If you are not keeping a constant dialogue with your colleagues in this manner, you could be losing out on an extremely useful source of advice. There is nothing to stop you starting an e-mail dialogue through the group address system. Contact your organisation's IT department for further ideas, which could include having your own ward manager's Web page based on frequently asked questions or even a discussion forum. A little time invested at the beginning goes a long way in terms of help and support in the future.

UTILISE THE PRACTICE DEVELOPMENT TEAM

Most health care organisations have some sort of professional or practice development team. They are usually directly managed and report to the director or deputy director of nursing. Their role is to work with all members of the health care team but particularly with ward managers, to facilitate improvements in clinical practice and spread good practice across the organisation. They support and advise all health care professionals and provide education and development not accessed through the universities (although they often link closely with local academic institutions).

The work of the practice development teams usually involves the following:

- Developing and implementing policies, procedures and best practice guidelines based on evidence.
- Provision of mandatory training, student and health care assistant (HCA) support and further clinical training.
- Dissemination of examples of good practice across the organisation.
- Assistance for staff to learn and take action from their experiences and patient feedback (e.g. from the complaints process).
- Improving staff access to the best evidence.

Try to involve the practice development team in any issue that involves changing or improving practice. If they are unable to give appropriate advice themselves, they will facilitate access to others who can. Some issues can be quite controversial, such as nil-by-mouth policies or nurse prescribing. The practice development team will help and guide you throughout the process. Even if you do not feel confident in the skills of your practice development team, it is best to keep them informed of any changes and improvements in your area to avoid duplication of any work in other departments.

They can also be an invaluable source of information. The team usually includes at least the following members.

Practice placement facilitator and practice educators

These people are usually employed in part or fully by the local universities to ensure that student nurses have appropriate placements and support during those placements. If you have any problems with students or problems with too many or too few students, these people should be your first port of call.

A health care assistant coordinator

An HCA coordinator is usually responsible for overseeing the training and development of HCAs throughout the organisation. They will also have links with external organisations/universities that deliver the diploma level 2 and 3 education programmes for HCAs.

A training and development coordinator

This person is usually responsible for coordinating the contracts with the local academic institutions and private education providers. Sometimes this role is incorporated into the deputy director of nursing role.

Nurses are also brought into the practice development team on secondments to facilitate the implementation of various national projects such as the Productive Series, safeguarding of vulnerable adults or dementia awareness. Together the team can be an invaluable source of advice and support. It's up to you to build up a good working relationship so you can call on them for advice in future situations.

ACTION POINTS

- Find out how to contact your organisation's solicitors both during and out of hours. Keep the details available in your ward office should the need arise.
- Find out who the main union officials are in your organisation; get to know them and add them to your network.
- Locate a copy of the course directory from your local university on the ward, so that you can access lecturers/experts in various subjects if required.
- Get to know your chaplaincy lead, add them to your network and ensure that all new recruits meet with them during their induction programme.
- Review the link nurse roles to ensure that each member of your team has no more than one. If necessary, prioritise with your team and set up different modes of communication to receive the necessary specialist information.
- Review your team's use of PALS and look for ways of improving the service you provide at ward level via appropriate information leaflets and staff education.
- Find out and familiarise yourself with *all* your organisation's performance indicators.
- Review all the policies and procedures on your ward, making sure they are up-to-date and easily accessible for all your staff.
- Take steps to ensure all members of your team are IT literate and make the most of resources available.
- Set up a group e-mail address on your computer to include all other ward managers within your organisation for access to support and advice.
- Get to know your practice development team and include them within your professional network.

References

Department of Health, 2003. NHS chaplaincy: meeting the religious and spiritual needs of patients and staff. Guidance for managers and those involved in the provision of chaplaincy-spiritual care. Online. Available: http://www.dh.gov.uk/assetRoot/04/06/20/28/04062028.pdf Feb 2012.

Dougherty, L., Lister, S., 2011. The Royal Marsden Hospital manual of clinical procedures, eighth ed. Blackwell, Oxford.

NHS Connecting for Health, 2011. Essential IT Skills programme. Online. Available: http://www.connectingforhealth.nhs.uk/systemsandservices/etd/eits Feb 2012.

NHS Litigation Authority, 2011. NHSLA Risk Management Standards. Online. Available: http://www.nhsla.com/RiskManagement/ Feb 2012.

Royal College of Nursing, 2011. RCN Direct online advice. Online. Available: http://www.rcn.org.uk/support/rcn_direct_online_advice Feb 2012.

UNISON, 2011. UNISON membership benefits: legal services. Online. Available: http://www.unison.org.uk/benefits/legal.asp.

QUESTION EXTERNAL DIRECTIVES

Sometimes other health care professionals or managers make decisions which adversely affect patient care or staff. Sometimes you may feel that you are pressured into making decisions which you do not feel are appropriate. The message here is don't always accept that others' decisions are the right ones.

Don't hesitate to challenge people just because they are more senior or are more knowledgeable in certain subjects than you. Trust your instincts. You are an experienced professional, and sometimes have more insight than they do. Often it is not what you say but how you say it that makes sure you are heard. If you find that certain performance indicators are reducing the standard of patient care or that undertaking audits is taking your staff away from patient care, you have a duty to speak up: 'You are personally accountable for actions and omissions in your practice and must always be able to justify your decisions' (Nursing and Midwifery Council (NMC) 2008).

IS ANOTHER LINK NURSE ROLE REALLY NEEDED?

Link nurses are a good way of maintaining links between the ward and various nurse specialists and people who are employed to enable the organisation to meet a particular quality indicator. The problem is that the number of nurse specialists and quality indicators is continually increasing. Some ward managers are now finding themselves in the position where the number of link nurse roles required is far greater than the number of staff they have on their team. Box 16.1 includes a small selection of the link nurse roles required from today's nurses.

PRIORITISE AND REPRIORITISE

Keep an up-to-date list of who is doing which link nurse role. Each time you are asked for another link nurse, don't automatically allocate the role to one of your staff. Get your team together first and reprioritise. Ask yourselves if this new link role is more important than the link roles you currently have. If it is, then identify which is the least important and drop it from your list. Find some other way of maintaining communication about the subject.

Try not to say to the person requiring the link roles that 'we are too busy and do not have the capacity to take on another role'. Be more specific. Show them the list of link roles you already have and explain why they are more important. Work out a compromise with them; it is in your best interests to maintain a good relationship with all nurse specialists.

Don't overburden your team with more than one link nurse role. Give each one the time and resources to gain full benefit from the work involved. The rest of your team and patients will also benefit.

BOX 16.1: A SMALL SELECTION OF THE LINK ROLES REQUIRED FROM TODAY'S WARD NURSES

Productive ward	Nutrition	Tissue viability
Infection control	Palliative care	Continence
Falls	Risk management	Education
Safeguarding	Manual handling	Child protection
Transfusion	Fire, health and safety	Pain
Medicines management	Diabetes	

GETTING THE MOST FROM THE LINK NURSE ROLE

The role of the link nurse usually entails the following:

1. Attending and contributing to regular meetings and study sessions.
2. Making information available to the rest of the team.
3. Keeping all patient and staff information sources up-to-date.
4. Helping to set and implement standards in the subject.
5. Evaluating and monitoring practice on the ward.
6. Identifying educational needs of the team.
7. Contributing to induction packages and staff teaching programmes.
8. Assisting with monitoring standards and auditing where necessary.
9. Identifying own educational needs and maintaining a high standard of professional competence in the subject area.

It takes time to be able to carry out these duties, so you should ascertain exactly how many hours per week or month will be required to undertake the role. Don't expect your staff to meet the demands of the link nurse role in their own time. It should be seen as a development opportunity, not a chore. Ensure the link roles are included in job descriptions and the budgeted staff establishment takes the role demands into account.

MONITOR EFFECTIVENESS OF THE LINK NURSE ROLE

Monitor how these link roles are enhancing patient care on your ward. Are they making a difference, or are the link nurses being used as administrators to do work not directly involving or affecting patient care within your own ward? Do this by making sure that link nurses report back to you regularly regarding the additional work they are undertaking.

HAS THE BED MANAGER CONSIDERED ALL OTHER OPTIONS?

Work with your bed manager. You may dread them coming on to your ward or ringing you up every 5 minutes, but they have to know what is going on everywhere and place patients in beds as soon as possible. They are under constant pressure and sometimes do not realise the pressures you have, especially those who do not have a clinical background.

EXPLAIN YOUR SITUATION CLEARLY

Never accept administrative decisions that compromise patient care. Your patients' welfare should always come first. Obviously you cannot refuse admissions in emergency situations when it is clear that there is nothing else available, but you must not routinely accept additional patients knowing that the quality of care that they or your existing patients receive will be compromised.

If you have said to the bed manager that you do not have the staff required to care for a new patient appropriately at that time but they still insist on sending the patient to you, you must explain clearly the implications of their decision, and put this in writing. It is usually preferable to do this by e-mail, sending a copy to your line manager and the appropriate duty manager.

WORK TOGETHER WITH THE OTHER WARD MANAGERS

Bed managers are used to nurses-in-charge saying that they do not have enough staff. It can get to the situation where the bed manager has to decide which short-staffed ward is worse off. The decision is sometimes based on the persuasiveness of the nurse-in-charge. It would help a lot more if you were to use your leadership skills of influencing and negotiating, to get all the wards to work together in these situations.

Use your close network with the other ward managers to create alternative solutions to these problems. You are the managers with the most clinical knowledge within the hospital and are probably in a better position to generate other options. The bed manager tends to work in isolation and does not have the knowledge and authority generated by a group of ward managers who communicate closely.

Working together as a group of ward managers alongside the bed manager will help reduce the problem of wards working against each other with regards to admissions. It may also help to stop some wards getting all the heavily dependent patients and makes sure that nurses get to care for patients in their specialty rather than struggling to nurse patients with illnesses of which they have little knowledge and who should probably be on another ward.

DON'T USE THE DAYROOM

For those who still have a dayroom, remember that caring for extra patients in the dayroom, in addition to those on the ward, is not usually costed within your staffing establishment and therefore should not be encouraged. The dayroom is not a waiting room to be used for those waiting to be admitted or discharged.

You cannot leave patients waiting for transport in the dayroom unless you have the appropriate staffing levels to monitor them. That is the role of the discharge lounge. Explain to the bed manager that you expect the bed to be available at a certain time, but will not accept a new patient until the previous patient has left.

If you are having your decision overturned by senior managers in your absence because of the pressure on waiting lists, make sure your staff book extra cover to look after the patients in the dayroom. Cost up the extra expense with your finance advisor and let your managers know in writing how much the decision is costing you. Unless you spell it out to managers and administrators, they may have no idea of the implications. Be specific: don't use vague terms, such as 'we are too busy' or 'we do not have enough staff' or 'it is affecting quality of care'. These phrases are heard every day and people become immune to such language. Use their language, such as 'we need an extra £2000 per month to cover staffing costs with patients waiting in the dayroom, which amounts to an extra £24000 per year'.

ARE YOU MANAGING A TEAM OF NURSES OR AUDITORS?

With the current national emphasis on quality indicators, virtually everything you do is audited. Improvements in both quality and quantity of care cannot be demonstrated unless regular audits are undertaken. However, auditing nursing care is currently taking up a lot of precious time which could be spent on nursing patients. In some situations you may find your team getting to the stage where they are spending more time auditing the care than administering the care itself. A situation may arise where auditing becomes the cause of a reduction in care standards in some areas. Hourly rounding is one example. If a nurse who has been allocated 10 patients has to spend each and every hour going round recording on forms what each patient says, what position they are in and whether they have a call bell nearby, her ability to assess, prioritise and administer appropriate care to those who really need it could be compromised.

FINANCIAL AND PROFESSIONAL IMPLICATIONS

Audits take time. Has the cost of this time been taken into consideration when working out your staffing establishment? How many staff hours does it take every week/month to fill in the various forms? It's worth taking some time to work it out with your finance advisor. Get together with your colleagues such as the other ward managers and work out how much time it is taking your staff to fill in all these audits, and therefore how much it is compromising patient care, especially when the information required from one audit overlaps with another. Together you can raise the issue with your director of nursing. With so many departments requiring information, senior managers do not always realise the impact that all these audits have on front-line workers. Some have even impacted on the nursing process. Admission documentation is an example where, in some areas, nurses have given up using an evidence-based nursing model with which to assess and plan care. In its place is a tick list of areas that require documenting for audit purposes.

AUDITS THAT ARE NOT PART OF CONTINUOUS QUALITY MONITORING

Consider first how the results are going to help you improve care if you are asked to undertake (yet another) audit on your ward. In the current climate of having to meet various quality indicators, taking on further audits is not helpful. If the audit is for someone else's benefit, then why are you doing all the work for them? What's in it for you? Don't undertake all audits without question. It is not your role to collect information for others. It is an administrator's role and most organisations have an audit department for this purpose. In addition, all audits must be registered with the audit department.

HAS YOUR LINE MANAGER QUESTIONED THE DECISION?

Don't always take 'no' for an answer from your line manager. If you have asked for something and your manager gives you a negative response, don't rant or rave, but don't stand down and accept their answer either if it's something that you really need. How do you know how hard they have tried on your behalf or even if they have tried at all? Before you accept a negative response, find out the facts (Table 16.1).

If you are unsatisfied with the response, don't go to the next manager up unless absolutely necessary. Undermining your own line manager can damage your future working relationship. Some line managers may not feel as passionately about the subject as you do and may not have tried very hard to get what you need. They may not fully understand what you want them to do or they may not know the right channels to go through.

Work with your manager to get the right results. Don't expect them to do things for you. When you receive a negative response and find they haven't tried hard enough, try again: 'Perhaps we could try a different approach?' or 'Perhaps if I find out some further information, we could put it forward as a business case?' Focus on using 'we' rather than 'you'; it's a less threatening approach and prevents unnecessary conflict.

DO SOME QUALITY INDICATORS ACTUALLY LOWER THE QUALITY OF CARE?

Quality indicators (such as those produced by the Commissioning for Quality and Innovation (CQUIN) and the Care Quality Commission (CQC) in England) are devised for the sole purpose of enhancing the quality of care. However, in order to meet certain quality indicators, some staff will accept the lowering of other aspects of care. For example, it has not been unknown for patients to go without appropriate first-line treatment in order to reach the performance indicator of reduced waiting times.

TABLE 16.1: How to find out the facts behind negative managerial responses

Negative response	Fact-finding response
'There's no money'	'Which budget are you referring to?' 'Was it put forward as part of this year's business plan?' 'What happened to the money that was granted for the project?'
'I've asked and you're not allowed'	'Who did you ask?' 'What are the reasons?' 'How did you present the case to them?'
'No, it's not possible for you to have any more staff'	'What are the reasons?' 'Have you discussed all the options with …?' 'Has it been included as part of next year's business plan?'

PUTTING PATIENT CARE FIRST

Quality indicators have been devised based on patient demands and the majority
are reasonable requirements that should be met. Unfortunately, some managers can
become so focused on meeting these indicators that they will do anything to reach
them, including the compromising of patient care. As a health care professional you
are bound by the code of conduct which puts the patients' welfare first when facing
any professional dilemmas. Unfortunately it can be difficult to challenge quality
indicators when putting patients first is the aim.

CHALLENGE UNREASONABLE QUALITY INDICATORS

Use your common sense. If you and your staff can see the quality of patient care
is being drastically affected, question what is happening. Make sure everyone
knows that clinical care is being compromised. Don't keep the knowledge within
your directorate. If a quality indicator is affecting others too, get them all involved.
Work together as a team to generate other ways of meeting the indicator that do
not compromise patient care. If you cannot do this, challenge the quality indicator
itself.

If you decide to challenge the indicator, make sure that you do this together with
the appropriate senior managers. You must look after yourself and your team. It
is not in your interests to be seen as 'difficult'. Your goal is to work with people
and generate enthusiasm to support each other in challenging the indicator and
suggesting alternative ways of improving care. It was not until the 'unnecessary
deaths' of at least 400 patients at Mid Staffordshire NHS Trust that the effects of
implementing the 4-hour A&E waiting time indicator were finally brought to light
(Francis 2010), and the target of reaching 98% was reduced. Following this inquiry,
the NMC issued guidance for nurses and midwives to 'speak up on behalf of people
in your care' (NMC 2010). It is part of your professional code of conduct to put
patients' welfare first (see p. 3 for more information on raising concerns).

ARE SENIOR MANAGERS AWARE OF THE IMPLICATIONS OF THEIR DECISION?

Senior managers (i.e. above band 8a) provide an invaluable service within health
care. They enable health care professionals to focus on their main area of expertise,
i.e. health care. However, there is one disadvantage in that many senior managers
have no experience in the delivery of hands-on health care. Without this experience
it is not easy to fully appreciate the pressures of dealing with unpredictable
workloads, constant and varying demands from sick and vulnerable patients
and the need to maintain clinical expertise in a continually advancing technical
environment.

Managing health care is a very different job from general management and,
unless they have been in a clinical role previously, it is difficult for senior managers
to understand the complexities of front-line patient care. There are bound to be

occasions where decisions are made which cause unintentional adverse effects in the delivery of health care. Some examples include the following:

1. The chairman who decides to give all staff within the organisation a day off for Christmas shopping in order to thank them for all their hard work that year. This sort of decision can be a nightmare for ward managers who are already struggling to cover their rosters and remain within budget (and have usually arranged something locally around the roster anyway).
2. The decision to instigate a recruitment freeze across the organisation. This is a common decision which in 24-hour wards results either in increasing expenditure due to the need to book extra agency and bank staff to meet minimum safety levels or in compromising patient safety. Ward managers are then required to cover both the original vacancies and the increasing sickness levels caused by the remaining staff trying to cover the extra patient caseload.
3. Nurses not being allowed to sleep on their (unpaid) breaks at night. Many staff who work nights are revitalised by having a short sleep on their break and evidence shows this to be the case (Fallis et al 2011). Some non-clinical managers may not appreciate that it could indeed be more dangerous if this is not allowed.

If decisions like this are being made and implemented without consultation in your organisation, don't accept it and moan and whinge among your peers. Ask yourself why you have not been involved in this decision. What can you do about it?

POINT OUT THE IMPLICATIONS OF THE DECISION

First, let the appropriate senior managers within the organisation know about the implications of their decision in writing. An e-mail can be less confrontational than a formal letter. Make sure you offer alternative solutions after consultation with your team and peers.

Be positive; you do not want to be labelled as the difficult one. Point out that you understand the predicament but that you and your staff believe there are valid alternative solutions which will reduce the risk of the negative effects that you have outlined. Offer to discuss this further with them if they so wish. Do not be defensive; you are part of the organisation and part of 'the management'.

Second, consider why you were not involved in this decision and what you can do so that you are involved next time. Make yourself known and widen your networks. You and your peers want to be consulted next time decisions like this need to be made. Find a way of ensuring that you are.

ARE CONSULTANT/SPECIALIST DECISIONS ALWAYS APPROPRIATE?

When an opinion has been requested by a specialist, always remember it is just that; an opinion. It does not mean that you have to do whatever is recommended. You and your staff know your patients better than most. Sometimes a specialist will come and give directions which are against your better judgement for that particular patient. A consultant may deem a patient fit for discharge whereas you know that the patient is not as independent as they seem. A nutritionist may recommend certain dietary restrictions for a patient that you are having problems getting any food down, let alone put on a special diet.

When you get to ward manager level, you should have gained the skills and confidence to be able to question consultant or specialist opinions, but your staff may not have this confidence. On the other hand, they may become overconfident and literally say what they think of the specialist's opinion without thinking of the long-term consequences on team relations.

TEACH YOUR STAFF THE ART OF DIPLOMACY

Your job is to maintain good relationships with all members of the multidisciplinary team but also to create an environment where your staff can challenge inappropriate clinical decisions. The key is to ensure that they are diplomatic in their questioning, and discourage any moaning and whingeing about the person's personality or behaviour afterwards. Be a role model and show your staff the most appropriate way to question decisions. For example:

1. Point out the positive: e.g. 'Yes. It would be nice if Mr X could go home today.'
2. Explain the problem briefly: e.g. 'But at the moment, he is still unable to get out of his bed unaided.'
3. Suggest a joint solution: e.g. 'Perhaps we can review this at the end of the week after 3 further days of rehabilitation.'

WHAT IF THE CONSULTANT/SPECIALIST IS WRONG BUT GOES AHEAD ANYWAY?

This rarely happens if you have spent time and effort in building up the relationship beforehand through the regular positive feedback approach (see p. 49). However, there may be occasions where a senior clinician is making decisions that are detrimental for your patient(s). If it is a one-off event, getting a second opinion is sometimes an option, but do be diplomatic, e.g. 'I called the ICU anaesthetist because the patient deteriorated right after you left and I was unable to get hold of you'.

However, you cannot keep doing this if the senior clinician continues with the same decisions. Under the terms of your professional code of conduct, you are obliged to take your concerns to a more senior level. Your line manager should be your first port of call, and if they are unable to solve the issue, then it is advisable to go to the director of nursing for professional advice and support. Your director of nursing should then take appropriate action. Each NHS organisation has a designated person to deal with such concerns. It is usually the director of nursing but may be one of the other directors. If you are unsure, your local trust 'whistleblowing' policy will have the name and contact details of that designated person.

REPORTING CONCERNS ABOUT ANOTHER HEALTH PROFESSIONAL

After the Bristol inquiry (where consultants continued to operate despite being told that their mortality rates were unusually high), every NHS organisation is now obliged to listen to their employees' concerns over others' clinical practice. The Bristol inquiry recommendations also set out quite clearly that 'The reporting of sentinel events must be made as easy as possible, using all available means of communication (including a confidential telephone reporting line)' (Kennedy 2001; Recommendation 113). Most NHS organisations now have an appropriate policy in place that ensures your concerns will be heard.

However, while we should try to be positive about the subject of accountability, it is worth considering first what could be the consequences before you or any of your staff decide to raise your concerns. It may be appropriate to abide by your code of conduct and take action that is best for your patients, but if you do decide to whistleblow, it is advisable to consider the worst case scenario. There is still a chance (albeit a small one since the implementation of formal policies on raising concerns) that you can become subject to defensive or ignorant behaviour from senior managers, so make sure that you prepare very carefully.

Keep copies of all documents, including e-mails. Any conversations not recorded on paper can easily be denied. Use e-mail rather than letters; letters may go unheeded. People can always deny they received a letter or say they forwarded it on but it got lost. See your trade union official for advice or contact the NMC. For more independent advice, you can contact Public Concern at Work (http://www.pcaw.co.uk). This is a charity set up in 1993 which is an independent authority on public interest whistleblowing. It offers free advice to people concerned about malpractice at work and who are unsure about whether or how to raise the matter.

DOES YOUR UNION STEWARD KNOW?

WHAT HELP ARE UNIONS?

Unions were set up to protect living standards and improve working conditions. As an individual, you do not always have the power to be able to negotiate with your board of directors or to make your voice heard. Union stewards have a stronger voice and usually meet regularly (every month) with board members to represent the views of the workforce.

Stewards from different unions meet together regularly as a formal group usually called the Joint Staff Side Committee (JSSC). This group liaises directly with the board of directors via another formal group called the Joint Consultative and Negotiating Committee (JCNC). The JCNC usually has at least one of the board directors attending each time. This is how local policies governing many aspects of your working conditions are agreed. Most JCNC meetings usually have to consist of 50% managers and 50% union stewards.

The role of the JCNC is to provide a forum for discussing or negotiating matters that affect employees, including issues stemming from:

- organisation change (e.g. ward closures, poor consultation)
- health and safety (e.g. unsafe working conditions)
- employee welfare (e.g. provision of catering facilities, withdrawal of changing facilities).

The committee also provides a mechanism for formal consultation regarding proposed future changes and serves to formally agree any changes and approve changes to terms and conditions for staff.

GETTING YOUR VOICE HEARD

Only recognised union stewards can attend the JCNC, so if you wish to raise any issue which involves or affects your staff and others within your organisation, you need to discuss it with your union steward first. They can raise the issue on your behalf. You may wish, for example, to raise concerns about a decision to reduce the canteen facilities for your night staff or a directive not to wear uniform outside the premises when no changing rooms are provided. These issues are wider than your remit as a ward manager and, as they affect other staff, they are probably better raised at the JCNC. There are certain situations where the union stewards' voices can be more effective than yours.

IS THE CHIEF EXECUTIVE AWARE OF WHAT IS HAPPENING?

The chief executive is responsible for ensuring that finance and quality are properly controlled. They are Accountable Officers, which means they are held responsible for ensuring that the organisation meets all its statutory and legal requirements.

STATUTORY DUTY FOR MAINTAINING QUALITY

Following the 1999 NHS Health Act, all chief executives now have a statutory duty to put and keep in place arrangements for monitoring and improving the quality of care provided to individuals. This means that your chief executive (along with the rest of the board) wants to make sure that all systems are in place within their organisation to maintain standards. If any part of the system is failing in any way, they do not want to be the last to know.

Don't always assume that the chief executive must know or that someone must have told them. It was found in 2010 that half the chief executives of trusts failing to comply with CQC standards of care were unaware of this fact (Santry 2010). Trust boards are always keen to keep informed about what is going on (or not going on) in the clinical area, particularly your director of nursing.

INAPPROPRIATE DECISIONS NEED TO BE HIGHLIGHTED

If the board or a senior manager has made a decision which adversely affects staff or patient care across the organisation, you may need to tell them directly. Don't moan and whinge about the effects; they may have no idea. It may be unintentional. Tell them. Most chief executives now have regular forums where they set aside an hour or so to meet with staff (anyone who wants to come along) and listen to their views. It's worth making use of these forums to raise and discuss any concerns that you have. You also have the option of sending an e-mail directly. A short e-mail saying 'I'm not sure whether anyone has realised but the new car park beside the outpatients department has no disabled access to bypass the steps which means that patients have not been able to attend their clinic appointments over the past 3 weeks since it was opened. I do apologise if this issue has already been raised but I have a feeling that we will not be the only department affected'.

It is unlikely that anyone would complain at receiving such an e-mail, but only send it if you have already tried the appropriate channels first, such as the facilities manager. The board director should be your very last option and definitely not the first port of call.

RELY ON YOUR OWN COMMON SENSE

No matter what the problem is, the number one principle of managing a ward should be to employ your common sense. There are many rules and regulations in health care to help you in making decisions. They were not made to be broken but there are times when the rulebook should not be taken literally. Good nurse managers will use their common sense and strive to uphold the intent of the rule rather than the actual rule itself.

Nothing beats the common sense approach learned through years of experience. It is common sense to:

- consult others before you make any decisions
- establish shared annual objectives with your team
- give consistent feedback to enable your team to grow
- take time to listen to your staff's concerns
- get to know all your staff well and treat them all equally
- take care of yourself and your health.

None of this is rocket science and you do not need to know all the management theories and models in order to manage a ward. In fact, most management theories and models have been included in this book. The jargon has just been removed. You remove jargon yourself every day by continually explaining concepts to patients in a language that they understand. I have just done the same for you.

Don't be afraid to challenge the system; just make sure you do so in a diplomatic and controlled manner. Sometimes people are so wrapped up in political correctness and afraid of doing the wrong thing that they do not trust their own judgement. Read and network widely to inform your decision making and learn from your experiences. They are worth no less than the experiences of others, so don't be afraid to trust your own instincts.

ACTION POINTS

- Together with your team, review and streamline your link nurse roles, particularly if there are any individuals who have more than one.
- Work together with the other ward managers and make joint decisions, particularly where decisions are concerned regarding bed management.
- Calculate the financial costs of all audit work in terms of staff time. Question all audits and, if possible, only undertake those that benefit your staff and patients directly.
- Don't always take your line manager's responses at face value. Question their actions and work with them for a better solution where appropriate.
- Find better ways of meeting quality indicators if the current way is detrimental to patient care. If there is no better way, question the indicator.
- Don't always assume that senior managers are aware of the implications of their decisions – find out.
- Don't always accept consultant or specialist decisions as being right, but be diplomatic when finding or implementing an alternative solution.
- Network closely with your organisation's senior union steward (the one who attends the JCNC).

References

Fallis, W.M., McMillan, D.E., Edwards, M.P., 2011. Napping during night shift: practices, preferences and perceptions of critical care and emergency department nurses. Crit. Care Nurse 31 (2). Online. Available: http://ccn.aacnjournals.org/content/31/2/e1.full Feb 2012.

Francis, R., 2010. Independent inquiry into care provided by Mid Staffordshire NHS Foundation Trust January 2005–March 2009, vol 1. HMSO, London.

Kennedy, I., 2001. Learning from Bristol: the report of the public inquiry into children's heart surgery at the Bristol Royal Infirmary 1984–1995. Online. Available: http://www.bristol-inquiry.org.uk/final_report.

Nursing and Midwifery Council, 2008. The code: Standards of conduct, performance, and ethics for nurses and midwives. London. Online. Available: http://www.nmc-uk.org.

Nursing and Midwifery Council, 2010. Raising and escalating concerns: guidance for nurses and midwives. Online. Available: http://www.nmc-uk.org/Documents/RaisingandEscalatingConcerns/Raising-and-escalating-concerns-guidance-A5.pdf Jan 2012.

Santry, C., 2010. CQC: half of trusts registered with conditions unaware of shortcomings. Health Serv. J. 8 Apr. Online. Available: http://www.hsj.co.uk/news/acute-care/cqc-half-of-trusts-registered-with-conditions-unaware-of-shortcomings/5013262.article.

Index

Notes: Page numbers followed by *f* indicate figures, *t* indicate tables, and *b* indicate boxes. *vs.* indicates a comparison or differential diagnosis